ADAPTIVE TAI CHI

Adaptive Tai Chi

AN ACCESSIBLE PRACTICE FOR EMPOWERING BODY AND MIND

ZIBIN GUO

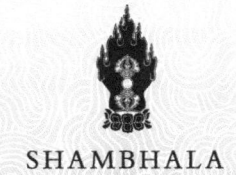

SHAMBHALA

Shambhala Publications, Inc.
2129 13th Street
Boulder, Colorado 80302
www.shambhala.com

9 8 7 6 5 4 3 2 1

First Edition
Printed in the United States of America

Shambhala Publications makes every effort to print on acid-free, recycled
paper.
Shambhala Publications is distributed worldwide by
Penguin Random House, Inc., and its subsidiaries.

Library of Congress Cataloging-in-Publication Data
Names: Guo, Zibin, 1961– author.
Title: Adaptive Tai Chi: an accessible practice for empowering body and
  mind / Zibin Guo.
Description: First edition. | Boulder: Shambhala, [2025] |
Identifiers: LCCN 2024046314 | ISBN 9781645472735 (trade paperback)
Subjects: LCSH: Tai chi. | Physical fitness for people with disabilities. |
  People with disabilities—Recreation.
Classification: LCC GV504 .G85 2025 | DDC 613.7/148155—dc23/eng/20241230
LC record available at https://lccn.loc.gov/2024046314

The authorized representative in the EU for product safety and compliance
is eucomply OÜ, Pärnu mnt 139b-14, 11317 Tallinn, Estonia, hello@
eucompliancepartner.com.

Contents

Introduction
Dancing in the Chair

THE LIGHT SWITCH

MY RELATIONSHIP WITH wheelchair Tai Chi Chuan started with an ordinary encounter shortly after I started graduate work at the University of Connecticut. One day I received a phone call from a man asking if I would be interested in offering him private Tai Chi Chuan lessons. Paul was a freelance writer who had read several volumes of the Chinese classics, including history and philosophy, and had also read about Tai Chi Chuan. "I have always wanted to learn the art of Tai Chi Chuan, and now the opportunity has come," he said over the phone. I was excited to share Tai Chi Chuan with someone who already knew so much about the ideas behind the practice and was eager to meet him.

After a brief conversation, we agreed to begin lessons in the basement office at his home the following week. He instructed me to go directly to the basement after entering the house and said that he would leave the front and basement door open for me. When we were about to hang up, he said, "By the way, I am blind." I was surprised. I had never taught Tai Chi Chuan to anyone who was blind. Sensing the hesitation in my response, he added, "I hope you don't mind teaching me. I am quite good at following verbal instructions." After a pause I replied, "Of course I do not mind."

On the day of our first lesson, I went to his house and opened the door to the basement. It was pitch black inside. I shouted, "I am here. Where is the light switch?" Paul shouted back, "Light switch? Why do we need light?" A few moments later, he turned the light on and greeted me with a humorous apology. But by then I was already enlightened. *He* did not need that assistive device, but I did.

Over the following weeks, we would spend the first part of each lesson discussing the American way of life, Chinese history, the philosophy of Daoism, Confucianism, and the ideas behind Chinese medicine. In addition to being a master Tai Chi Chuan instructor, I am a professor of medical anthropology with a deep interest in classical Chinese literature. Watching the way he elegantly moved his arms and body during these conversations, I often forgot that he did not have sight.

One day I asked him which aspect of Tai Chi Chuan attracted him the most. Without hesitation he replied that it was its "flow." I asked him why he found flow attractive. He replied, "Don't we all?" He smiled and said he knew exactly what I was asking. "You asked why a blind guy like me finds flow attractive, right?" The way he put it, "a blind guy like me," made me feel awkward. He laughed and said, "Why do I find the flow attractive? Because there is hardly any in my world." I felt I knew what he meant but did not know how to respond.

Unfortunately, the lessons did not continue for much longer. We decided to call it quits after Paul fell a few times during practice. At the end of our last lesson, Paul said, "Don't worry. The few moves you have taught me are enough to enjoy." I was disappointed that I did not know how to share the art of flow in Tai Chi Chuan with Paul, who loved it so much.

It was a short encounter, but meeting Paul offered me a lasting gift. Our seemingly ordinary exchange about the light switch had given me extraordinary insights. It challenged my perceptions of "normal" and "ability" and directed my thoughts to how we tend to classify and label human body conditions and abilities. For example, why do some assistive devices, such as lights, "normalize" some conditions but not others? I was particularly struck by Paul's statement that there is hardly any flow in his world. It was not until later, during my medical anthropology studies, that I realized that the world Paul called "his" is the same as mine. It is also the same world that developed Tai Chi and figured out how to empower our limitations and transform challenges through the flow of mind and body.

FIELDWORK

Shortly after meeting Paul, I enrolled in the PhD program in medical anthropology at the University of Connecticut. I was inspired to study the social and cultural forces that shape our perceptions of health problems and the practices we develop to make sense of and deal with them. The program gave me both a theoretical and methodological foundation for understanding health issues. It was a perfect complement to my longtime passion for Tai Chi and my interest in applying the principles and methods of the traditional healing arts to develop socially and culturally sound intervention programs that meet the needs of contemporary people.

In May 1992 I moved to Flushing, New York, to begin my dissertation field research. Funded by the National Center for Health Statistics, my fieldwork focused on examining the social and cultural factors affecting health-care management among two groups of elderly Asian Americans. To get a firsthand understanding of the needs of these immigrants, I quickly became immersed in their community life. During my research, I served as a translator for their hospital visits, helped them enroll in Medicaid, participated in their family and social festivities, took part in a Bible study group, volunteered at senior centers, and even sang karaoke at their birthday parties.

Through these participatory research activities, I established close bonds with many individuals. I learned a great deal about their daily challenges in dealing with health-related issues too. I was inspired by their spirit and efforts at achieving physical well-being and peace of mind, despite the abundant disadvantages and obstacles they faced in obtaining access to health care: limited financial means, language barriers, differing cultural assumptions about health and illness, and cultural stereotypes and discrimination by mainstream health-care providers.

After I was awarded my PhD in 1994, I joined a multidisciplinary research team at Harvard Medical School and participated in a National Institute of Aging longitudinal study exploring the social and cultural factors influencing the recognition of and response to dementia-related symptoms among caregivers from several ethnic groups in the Boston area. During three years of ethnographic research, I learned a great deal about the dynamics of disease labeling and its power to affect individual and social perceptions of the "diseased" body. The reluctance to accept dementia-related labels within a few minority communities did not necessarily indicate a complete repudiation of a dementia-related diagnosis. Rather, the disassociation of such symptoms from clinical labels that normalized mental decline often helped the elderly and their family members to better cope with the symptoms.

My graduate and postgraduate work in medical anthropology and applied anthropology gave me a fresh, holistic perspective to understand the social and cultural dynamics of the body and mind. Through the lens of social and cultural adaptations, I deeply understood that the historically beneficial effects of Tai Chi Chuan practice on our holistic well-being are attributed to its focus on strengthening the body through empowering the mind. The power of Tai Chi practice is timeless. It can remedy a whole range of social and population issues and can be applied to transform a perceived vulnerability into a source of strength.

This training and experience gave me the confidence to develop a form of adaptive Tai Chi Chuan. Now people like Paul and thousands of others who live with a range of abilities would be empowered by developing a flowing mind.

A Flowing Nature

I used to have an office on the third floor of a building at the center of a university campus. A big, wide window overlooked the university center, downtown, and the distant mountains. Many visitors commented on the beautiful view as soon as they entered the office. Over the years I would randomly ask why they thought the view was attractive. Everyone described their impressions differently, but they mostly said the view was "flowing," "dynamic," "tranquil," "harmonious," "naturalistic," "a mix of natural and modern elements," and "pretty."

We all enjoy viewing natural landscapes. Sweeping vistas, dramatic rock formations, colorful foliage, and calmly flowing mountain streams can be captivating and awe-inspiring. It is interesting that the beauty of nature seems to be all about its biodiversity and the interplay among diverse elements that create dynamic patterns and flows. What if we focused on comparing objects in nature—for example, what if we favored giant trees over smaller ones, or looked down at a trickle of a stream and faulted it for not being a raging river? We would never apply that kind of judgment to nature. But don't we classify our bodies according to their evident physical traits, the composition of various parts, and their social abilities?

Flow is the natural way to transform a perceived vulnerability into beauty. Just as when we view a natural landscape, in Tai Chi Chuan the graceful mind-centered flowing body movement not only makes practitioners feel graceful, but it also generates power. To engage in flowing movement, all body parts, short or long, strong or weak, must work together as one dynamic system without partiality.

VULNERABILITY IS A SOURCE OF POWER

I began practicing external martial arts, including Northern Shaolin, Chaquan, and various weapon forms, at a very young age. Inspired by my teacher, Master Xue-Xi Fan, an accomplished and respected external martial artist in China, I dreamed of becoming a great martial artist like him. However, I badly injured my back during a sparring practice with my martial-arts brothers. Doctors told me that I had to stop practicing any movements that would stress the back if I wanted to have a healthy back for the rest of my life. I was desperate and depressed. My master told me that I could keep my dream alive if I practiced Tai Chi Chuan. I had a bias against Tai Chi Chuan at that time and had little knowledge about its hidden power. However, eventually I decided to give it a try.

One early summer morning I went to a local park to meet Master Gongwei Xu, a respected internal martial artist in Nanjing. When I arrived at the park, Master Xu had just finished leading a group of students of all ages in a routine of Chen-style Tai Chi Chuan. Master Xu was in his early seventies and had a slender build and a kind smile; his eyes had a compassionate yet resolute gaze. After gently shaking my hand and welcoming me, he asked how much I knew about Tai Chi Chuan. "Nothing at all," I honestly replied. He probably sensed my lack of excitement and decided to give me a hands-on learning experience about the gentle power of Tai Chi Chuan. He pulled his left foot one small step back, forming a bow stance, and said, "Place your hands on my chest and push me as hard as you can." I could not believe what I heard, so I asked, "What did you say?" Master Xu gently repeated his request, looking at me gently and invitingly. I thought it was a ridiculous request. Even though my back had been injured a few months ago, I was still young and capable of using my body, having more than a decade of martial-arts practice and competition experience. I truly believed he did not realize how fast I could throw punches and kicks. He looked at me and said again, "I am ready." A dozen students gathered around and cheered us on. I could tell they were looking forward to seeing what happened next. I kept telling myself, "Do not do it, do not hurt the old man." Of course, in the mind of an eighteen year old, anyone over thirty was considered old. And he asked again, with a more commanding tone. I thought I had to do something symbolic to get this ritualistic test over with. So I walked to Master Xu, placed my palms against his front shoulders, and gently pushed, only using 20 percent of my power. Of course he did not move at all. He looked at me and asked, "Did you have breakfast yet?" Everyone around us laughed. I felt my face begin to burn and I was embarrassed and not happy. He looked at me and said, "Now you are ready. Hurry up, give a real push."

I put my palms on his shoulders and adjusted my stance. I pushed, using 80 percent of my strength. The moment I pushed him, I felt that his body was as weak as a soft pillow being pushed away. I immediately thought, "He is going to get hurt." Before I could finish my thought, however, I realized that my body was falling backward, and then I rolled on the ground a few meters away. Sitting on the grass, stunned, I turned around trying to figure out what had happened. Master Xu still stood at the same spot. That was the day I began to learn Tai Chi Chuan with Master Xu.

As you'll see, I've used a maxim throughout this book that is central to the art of Tai Chi Chuan: "A force of four ounces deflects one thousand pounds." This saying expresses ancient wisdom on our relative physical capabilities and the immeasurable potential of our minds. In the art of Tai Chi Chuan, the body's power is not determined by bodily conditions. Instead, our bodies are empowered through the mind. A calm and flowing mind not only unifies our body parts, turning them into a gently flowing system, but also enables the flowing system to create a soft and embracing force (of four ounces) to harness one thousand pounds of external challenges. Guided by the principles of Tai Chi Chuan, the practice transcends the narrow concept of physical ability as brute force or dominance to cultivate the "ultimate," which is unified, gentle, flowing, invisible, and immeasurable, like water.

Therefore Tai Chi Chuan is fundamentally an art of transforming the "weak," "vulnerable," and "disabled" into a source of force through flowing, gentle, simple, and unified body movements. The process of cultivating this force not only provides tremendous therapeutic benefits to all but also empowers us to find flow through the rigidities of our social worlds.

ASSISTIVE DEVICES, BEAUTY, AND ABILITY

The aspiration of applying wheelchair Tai Chi Chuan to make the practice of Tai Chi Chuan accessible for people like Paul and to demonstrate their ability creating power and beauty was inspired by watching a figure-skating event. Like Tai Chi Chuan, figure skating embodies grace, flow, harmony, change, creativity, mastery, emotion, and mind. One evening during the Winter Olympics I watched TV, captivated by the world's top skaters gliding across the ice, jumping and spinning, and flowing from one move to the next like dancers on ice. I imagined practicing Tai Chi Chuan in a wheelchair and flowing with the rolling wheels, just like a skated figure on the ice. Assisted devices like ice skates and wheelchairs are transformed into tools for creating power and beauty when the devices and body movements are integrated into one flowing movement.

Wheelchair Tai Chi Chuan is a perfect illustration of the very idea that gave birth to the art of Tai Chi Chuan. Tai Chi Chuan embodies the ancient wisdom of empowerment, which in Tai Chi Chuan goes beyond a particular body condition and functionality and is concentrated on a state of mind that is tranquil, clear, unified, flowing, and fluid. This state of mind can embrace all the body's abilities and transform them into a unified, gentle, flowing force.

Synthesizing the flowing motions of the wheelchair with the body's movements enables flowing body movements that lift the practitioner's spirit and provide a sense of expanded space and mobility. It also makes the wheelchair a source of power for the body, transforming disability into ability.

THE BENEFITS OF WHEELCHAIR TAI CHI CHUAN PRACTICE

To get a deeper understanding of the research literature on disability and rehabilitation, I worked with people who use wheelchairs and talked to rehabilitation health-care providers, including physical, occupational, and therapeutic-recreation therapists. This gave me insights into the shared health needs and challenges facing individuals with ambulatory disabilities.

Through this process, it became evident that a wheelchair Tai Chi Chuan program tailored to physical conditions and needs would also offer an ideal option for engaging in physical fitness. Here are a few key points:

1. According to rehabilitation research, many people with disabilities are reluctant to participate in physical activities because they fear that movements may cause pain or injury. When seated, all stress on the body muscles and joints is minimized, making the mind and body more relaxed and at ease.

2. In this environment, practitioners feel more comfortable gently rotating the lower back and hip area in a wide range of motion, which provides necessary fitness conditioning and boosts circulation.

3. The wide range of gentle, slow movements (body-engaged contracting and expanding circular flow, integrated with deep breathing) promotes blood and Qi circulation. This not only promotes healing to muscle and joint injuries but also massages the organs, improving their functionality.

4. Each circular movement in Tai Chi Chuan represents a specific principle and method of embracing and redirecting an external force, and performing these movements requires gentle, slow motion. Practicing these movements can empower and transcend the body's limitations, thus encouraging further practice.

5. A key feature of this program is that it integrates wheelchair motion (the rolling and turning of the chair) with the dynamic, gentle, and flowing movements of Tai Chi Chuan in a way that lifts the spirit and gives practitioners a sense of commanding space, thus transforming an assistive device—the wheelchair—into a tool for creating flow and beauty.

6. Wheelchair Tai Chi Chuan is accessible, low cost, and safe. It can be done anywhere without additional equipment and with few space constraints.

DEVELOPING THE THIRTEEN POSTURES OF WHEELCHAIR TAI CHI CHUAN

Conventional Tai Chi Chuan movements were developed by early martial artists and not all movements would suit people with an ambulatory challenge. To create a wheelchair program that can be therapeutic, empowering, and transformative, the principles of Tai Chi Chuan movements must be integrated with practical wheelchair use.

To be sure that the movements selected for the wheelchair Tai Chi Chuan program would suit people with ambulatory challenges, I spent a lot of time sitting in a wheelchair and maneuvering it around my home while practicing various Tai Chi Chuan movements to experience their effect on my body and mind. I reflected on how they could best flow with the forward roll and turn of the wheelchair. I realized that some movements would allow a more extensive range of motion in my lower back and hip without losing my balance than others. Practicing specific movements made me feel more powerful and energized, providing me with a sensation of infinite space despite being in a wheelchair.

For optimal therapeutic results, I chose thirteen movements from Yang- and Chen-style Tai Chi Chuan based on the following considerations:

1. Movements best suited to practice in wheelchairs.
2. Movements that allow an extensive range of motion for the lower back and hips.
3. Movements that promote rotation and a range of motion for the torso, lower back, shoulders, arms, and wrists.
4. Movements that help promote upper-body mobility and internal circulation.
5. Movements that combine vertical and horizontal circles to create a sense of infinite space between the mind and the body.
6. Movements that can be best integrated with wheelchair motions.
7. Movements that help increase a practitioner's sense of empowerment.

WHEELCHAIR TAI CHI AS A METAPHOR

We all have disabilities within given social contexts and we are all vulnerable. Recognizing this vulnerability, and the fluid nature of our abilities and body conditions, can be a source of courage, creativity, and joy in our life journeys. This understanding is the basis of the transformative power of Tai Chi Chuan, particularly adaptive Tai Chi Chuan.

Recognizing human vulnerability and transforming it into opportunity inspired the creation of Tai Chi Chuan. Over the centuries, this positive focus not only played a role in transforming vulnerability into empowerment but also became a powerful metaphor for our innate connection with nature when all states of being are part of transformative flow. The adaptive Tai Chi Chuan programs introduced in this book show us how we can empower our minds and bodies regardless of our abilities, building confidence and altering our outlook.

Since the debut of the wheelchair Tai Chi Chuan program at the 2008 Paralympics and the subsequent successful implementation of adaptive and inclusive Tai Chi Chuan in various vulnerable populations, this unique therapeutic model has garnered global recognition and has resonated with communities worldwide, from disability and human-rights organizations to rehabilitation medicine and mental-health groups, inner-city youth empowerment groups, aging and health forums, and cancer support groups. The program has been invited to present at numerous national and international professional organizations and conferences, including the International Tai Chi Symposium, the American Therapeutic Recreation Association Conference, the Society for Disability Studies Annual Conference, the American Physical Therapy Annual Conference, the American Anthropological Association Annual Conference, the Spinal Cord Injury Research Conference, the Mayo Clinic, the World Congress of the International Society of Physical and Rehabilitation Medicine, the International Society of Psychiatric-Mental Health Nurses Annual Conference, the European Congress of Physical and Rehabilitation Medicine, the American Psychiatric Nursing Conference, the United States Public Health Services Scientific Symposium, the National VA Wheelchair Games Education Program, and the UNESCO-ICM (International Centre of Martial Arts).

The worldwide embrace of this program not only underscores the broad applications and creative implications of the adaptive and inclusive Tai Chi Chuan program but also gives me the courage to write this book, with a sincere hope that it will provide you with new ideas and approaches to making life more interesting and enjoyable.

THE STRUCTURE OF THIS BOOK

Part 1 of this book contains four chapters on the wisdom traditions of Tai Chi Chuan. The first three chapters offer a survey of how Tai Chi emerged, the social contexts that transformed it from an applications-focused martial art to a healing-focused art, and the principles that make it a timeless treasure. Chapter 4 tells the story of developing the wheelchair program to the Paralympics stage and making it a therapeutic, interventive, recreational, and self-care modality for people with all body conditions, including persons with physical and psychological challenges or concerns, inner-city youth, veterans with disabilities, healthcare providers, and elderly populations.

Part 2 contains five chapters on the practice of inclusive Tai Chi. I include five complete practice modalities with photo illustrations of this seven-posture inclusive Tai Chi Chuan program: chapter 5 is the wheelchair modality, chapter 6 is the standing modality, chapter 7 is the simple walking modality, chapter 8 is the seated modality, and chapter 9 is the single-movement modality. The instructions in each chapter provide you with step-by-step practice illustrations and my interpretation of Tai Chi Chuan principles and their universal benefits.

As you read this book, you'll notice that the words "adaptive" and "inclusive" are used somewhat interchangeably. In the context of this book, "adaptive" refers to making the practice suitable for a particular body condition, such as the wheelchair modality. "Inclusive" refers to the program's design, the five practice modalities that are variations on one seven-posture Tai Chi Chuan sequence that can accommodate all individuals, regardless of their physical or psychological challenges and needs.

I'd love to hear from you if you have any questions about your practice or if you need any additional information about this program or the video illustrations. I'd be happy to direct you to the source.

Stand like a tree, sit like a mountain, flow like a river.

—Zibin Guo, August 2024

PART ONE   Philosophy

1

Learning from Nature

"Look deep into nature, and then you will
understand everything better."
—ALBERT EINSTEIN

Throughout human history, many thinkers across world cultures were inspired by the interplay between humans and the natural world. From Heraclitus and Plato to Lao-Tzu and Confucius, ancient philosophers advocated the idea that humans are a part of nature and are interconnected with the ever-changing natural world. However, because of their varying geographical, cultural, social, and historical contexts, they approached these relationships and their implications for human social life differently. For example, early Western thinkers often emphasized human domination over nature and using natural resources to benefit humans. On the other hand, early Eastern cultures advocated harmony with the natural world to best empower humans and sustain society.

Most relevant for our purposes is the emergence of the concept of *Tai Chi* in the Western Zhou period (1050–771 B.C.E.). *Tai Chi* (太极, *Taiji*) refers to the "supreme ultimate" or "great ultimate," a state in which an immeasurable amount of power can be cultivated through the interplay of opposites. It is said that the state of Tai Chi emerged from Wu Chi (无极, *Wuji*), a state perceived as primordial and undifferentiated potential. The emergence of Tai Chi as a philosophical construct epitomizes early thinkers' efforts to achieve an organized and harmonized social life through the *Dao* (道, *Tao*), or "the Way" of nature.

THE BIRTH OF TAI CHI CHUAN

The Zhou dynasty ruled ancient China for some eight centuries. After years of moral decline and corruption within the elite classes, internal revolts, rebellions, invasions, economic disparities, and social changes, the Zhou dynasty came to an end. The dynasty transformed into the Eastern Zhou in the Spring and Autumn and Warring States periods (771–221 B.C.E.), an era of great social chaos and enlightenment.

As the ancient Chinese people witnessed the long-running and once-powerful Zhou dynasty in a state of collapse, their hopelessness, anxiety, and agony intensified. A period called "the Hundred Schools of Thought" emerged, which produced schools of philosophy and classics meant to remedy the crisis and save the dynasty. These classics, which provided enlightenment and birthed the art of Tai Chi Chuan (太极拳, *Taijiquan*), include books familiar to contemporary audiences: the *I Ching*, or *Book of Changes* (易经, *Yijinguyi*); the *Daodejing* (道德经, *Tao Te Ching*); and the *Yellow Emperor's Classic of Internal Medicine* (黄帝内经, *Huangdi Neijing*).

THE *I CHING* AND SOURCES OF HARMONY

Clae Waltham wrote in the introduction of an English translation of the *I Ching*, "It has been called the oldest extant writings in the world, China's unique heritage, and a great treasure for all mankind."* The *I Ching* is considered to be one of the most influential sources for traditional Chinese social and cultural developments.

The *I Ching* asserts that humans are a part of nature and that to understand the deeper meaning of changes in the social world, we need to understand the *Dao* of changes in the natural world. Although the scope of nature's changes are too immense to comprehend, there are patterns that we can recognize. The *I Ching* proposes that natural changes tend to follow specific patterns:

1. The natural world exists because of the constant motion and change that transforms its state from Wu Chi to Tai Chi.
2. The changes in the natural world are all-encompassing, affecting all aspects of natural phenomena, activities, and human lives.
3. All motions of change flow from one form (imbalance) to the other (balance) in a repetitive cycle. The end of one circle is the beginning of the next.

*Clae Waltham, *I Ching: The Chinese Book of Changes* (New York: Ace Books, 1969).

4. The natural world maintains equilibrium through such a flowing change.

5. Change defines not only all lives in the natural world but also the process of generating energy and power to sustain the natural world and all lives within the natural world, including humans.

6. The constantly evolving natural world is driven by energies created by interactions and mutual transformations of two great opposing forces that are metaphorically named *yin* and *yang*.

7. *Yin* and *yang* originate from an indescribable state of being that possesses supremely immeasurable power and ability, and whose limits are intangible. The state of being, or "ability," is called the *Dao* or *Tai Chi*.

FOUR OUNCES VS. ONE THOUSAND POUNDS

The concept of *Dao* has been interpreted in different contexts throughout history. The terms *Dao* and *Tai Chi* describe a state that gives rise to all activities and energies. *Tai* (太) implies that something is grand or supreme in capability. *Chi* (极, *ji*) refers to limits, boundaries, or poles. Furthermore, the word *Tai* is formed from two Chinese characters: big (大) and the symbol for something as small as a dot (、). *Tai Chi*, therefore, conveys the sense of the "supreme ultimate," a formless state of being that can be as small as a dot yet give birth to the immeasurable power that drives the changes of all things, as in the previously noted maxim "A force of four ounces deflects one thousand pounds."

The *I Ching* gives us a philosophical framework for seeing that the cyclical changes in the natural and social worlds are interconnected and governed by the same Dao. Change is the driving force of life and the mechanism for maintaining equilibrium. So where exactly is the Dao or Tai Chi, the supreme ultimate, in humans? The Chinese scholar Ming Dong Gu wrote that the "Dao/Taiji may be seen as standing for the totality of the rationally structuring process of the mind."* Just as the Dao functions in the natural world, the weightless mind in humans can generate immeasurable power to navigate, regulate, and overcome the seemingly immense weight of formidable challenges and changes.

*Ming Dong Gu, "The Theory of the Dao and Taiji: A Chinese Model of the Mind," *Journal of Chinese Philosophy* 36, no. 1 (2009): 159.

In short, the *I Ching* became the first classical Chinese philosophy text to lay the foundation for mind-focused intellectual inquiry and cultural traditions. The wisdom that is revealed through nature has shaped Chinese philosophy, medicine, health practice, and martial arts, including Tai Chi Chuan.

THE *DAODEJING* AND TRANSFORMATION

The second influential text to lay the foundation for the birth and development of Tai Chi Chuan was the *Daodejing*, the classic text on the way of empowerment. *Daodejing* suggests that social disharmony is a consequence of losing sight of the Dao, as people become obsessed with rigidly defined social positions and material possessions (manifestations). Striving for material things may disorient people's minds from the Dao and weaken their ability to navigate life and its challenges. "Ever desireless, one can see the mystery, ever desiring, one can see the manifestation," as stated in the beginning of the book.* Therefore, to overcome these challenges, one must empower one's mind by learning from the Dao and the way of nature.

The *Daodejing* makes two key statements: what makes the natural world everlasting is that all changes follow the Dao, and what makes the Dao supremely ultimate is that it is nameless, desireless, and formless. It exists everywhere and flows like water. Dao is indescribable not because of its complexity but because of its simplicity. And because of these features, Dao acts effortlessly, promoting the changes and transformations between the yin and yang of all things in nature—again, the idea that four ounces of power can move one thousand pounds.

Opposites abound in nature: day and night, the four seasons, tall and short, cold and hot, and strong and weak. The relationship between these opposites is neither antagonistic nor tangible. The opposites are mutually inclusive and transform to and from each other like a fast-moving river. Through this lens, formlessness, effortlessness, simplicity, and fluidity are the qualities that make the Dao the supreme ultimate in the natural world.

To bring harmony and sustainability to life, one must cultivate a mind

*Lao Tsu, *Tao Te Ching*, trans. Gia-Fu Feng and Jane English (New York: Vintage Books, 1997): 1.

as fluid as water, as centered and calm as the Dao in the natural world, to navigate life's complexity. The *Daodejing* states:

> What (mind) is firmly established cannot be uprooted . . .
> Stiff and unbending is the principle of death.
> Gentle and yielding is the principle of life.
> The hard and stiff will fall.
> The gentle and fluid will overcome.

NEIJING AND THE INTEGRATION OF MIND AND BODY

Understanding and finding remedies for disease, injuries, and sickness has been one of humankind's the greatest challenges. *Neijing* (the *Yellow Emperor's Classic of Internal Medicine*), an ancient Chinese medical text written during the Warring States period, exemplifies such extraordinary efforts.

Neijing views the mind as an integrated part of the body. Social behaviors and physical conditions are products of our state of mind and mirror the condition of the mind. In *Neijing*, the distressed mind, expressed in unbalanced emotions, can disrupt the harmonious relationship of *yin* and *yang* in the body, contributing to illness. As the *Neijing* stated, "They (the sages) were tranquilly content in nothingness and true vital force accompanied them always; their vital (original) spirit was preserved within; thus, how could illness come to them?"* To remedy illness, the *Neijing* prescribes that we first heal and empower the mind by following nature's way. A calm, fluid, and engaged mind transforms the mind into the supreme ultimate, a state of possibility. This state of mind is the foundation for empowering the body by cultivating the flow of Qi within the body. Qi also guides human behavior and social engagement. In short, the Dao drives everlasting changes by embracing and unifying all forces.

These three foundational classics of Chinese philosophy—the *I Ching*, the *Daodejing*, and the *Neijing*—offer invaluable and timeless wisdom to promote and sustain social and cultural well-being based on the

---

*Ilza Veith, trans., *The Yellow Emperor's Classic of Internal Medicine* (Baltimore, MD: The Williams & Wilkins Company, 1949).

understanding that humans are integrated into the natural world and the natural world is the source of human empowerment and well-being. They also laid the foundation for the developments of natural healing practices, traditional Chinese medicine, and the martial arts, including Tai Chi Chuan.

Wu Chi: The original, primordial state of nothingness before Tai Chi. For example, a calm mental state after meditation.

Tai Chi: Transformed from Wu Chi and giving birth to the polarization (yin and yang) of all matter. In this state, the interplay of opposites creates immeasurable energies that fuel and govern the growth and flow of all life.

Yin and Yang: A metaphorical concept that implies the dual nature of all matter, which consists of two opposing but complementary forces. The interplay of these opposites creates unified energy that sustains life and governs its trajectory.

Qi: A multifaceted concept symbolizing the invisible and flowing nature of all energies created through the interplay of opposites. In the context of traditional Chinese medicine, Qi of various types is seen as the source and the driving force for the physiological activities of all body parts and organs.

EMPOWERING HUMANS BY IMITATING ANIMAL MOVEMENTS

In premodern times, illness and other misfortunes were often explained and managed within a spiritual conceptual framework. Many people perceived the way of the natural world to be mysterious and magical, ruled by invisible spiritual energies. They felt the consequences of these energies but could not control them, which triggered feelings of admiration and fear. *Shen Nong's Herbal Classics*, a foundational text in traditional Chinese medicine, and others, provided a different outlook: health and well-being are influenced by what we do and eat, and nature is the source of empowerment. Inspired by this behavioral model of well-being, people began to explore and imitate the movements of animals with admirable qualities to empower the body.

During the Han dynasty (206 B.C.E.–220 C.E.), an exercise called "The Art of Guiding and Stretching" (导引术, *Dao Yin Shu*) became popular. The exercise combines breath regulation (Qi Gong) and animal-like movements to strengthen the body and ward off disease. The well-known physician Hua Tuo (华佗, 141–208 C.E.) created a set of varied physical movements and breathwork called "Five Animals Play" (五禽戏, *Wu Qin Xi*), which imitates tiger, deer, bear, ape, and crane movements to regulate the circulation of Qi and blood, nourish the internal organs, and strengthen muscles and bones. These creative exercises transformed classical philosophical concepts into practices based on the interconnectedness between human well-being and the way of the natural world. The human body and mind could go from ordinary to extraordinary. These two healing exercises, developed more than two thousand years ago, have been continuously practiced worldwide to the present day, benefiting many.

The integration of animal movements into martial-arts practices underscores how one's ability, or power, and the condition of one's body are purely relative. For example, tigers and praying mantises are very different species, but each uses its distinct skills to overcome challenges in its complex and harsh environment. Animal movements are naturally fluid, varied, precise, balanced, effective, and graceful. By making a small circle with its forelimbs, a praying mantis successfully traps and blocks an opponent's strikes. A snake uses slow, coiling movements to quickly strike and subdue its prey. A crane elegantly opens its wings to signal a threat and it beaks its opponent. A duck effortlessly uses its grounded body to fend off a predator.

People recognized that mimicking their movements would enhance their martial-arts abilities by giving them a wider range of techniques for different situations. Mimicking animal movements would also allow humans to foster a mental connection with animals and the natural world, further empowering their bodies and movements. Today, these movements are categorized as "animal styles" in Chinese martial arts.

These innovations enabled people to transform the imperfect human body into a formidable force that could be primed to overcome any challenge. These practices embodied ancient wisdom and healing principles, which transformed them into self-empowerment practices.

Mimicking animals' natural movements confirmed what the ancient philosophers revealed about the Dao of the natural world: overcoming conflict is possible through fluid, unifying, redirecting, and transformative movements instead of rigid, forceful, and confrontational ones. A new martial-arts school, the internal martial arts, was born. Unlike conventional or external martial arts, which relies on physical strength, power, and speed to defeat opponents, internal martial arts uses the mind to focus one's body movements to redirect the opponent's power.

Mastering the internal martial arts takes much longer than the external martial arts. As my first martial-arts teacher, Master Xue-Xi Fan, said, "I can teach you how to use a staff in a month, but it takes a lifetime to learn how to use the mind to defeat your opponent."

For a long time, the internal martial arts were practiced mainly among small groups of martial artists, including Daoist martial artists and healing practitioners, and many were scholars of the *I Ching*, the *Daodejing*, and traditional Chinese medicine. These practitioners continued to incorporate the key concepts, ideas, and methods from these classic texts and over time transformed the internal martial arts into a mind-centered method of body engagement that laid the foundation for the modern system of Tai Chi Chuan.

THE BIRTH OF MODERN TAI CHI CHUAN

The term *Tai Chi Chuan* integrates two concepts. *Tai Chi* refers to the ultimate supreme, a state of being that can give birth to immeasurable power. *Chaun* (拳, *Quan*) means "fist" or "movement." Tai Chi Chuan refers to the practice that cultivates a state of mind that produces immeasurable power.

Tai Chi Chuan emerged as a distinctive form of internal martial arts during the late Ming dynasty (1368–1644 C.E.). The debate over its origin is ongoing, mainly because Tai Chi Chuan movements were referred to by different names for a long time. However, the first modern form of Tai Chi Chuan, with systematically developed illustrations, principles, methods, and applications, was created by Chen Wangting (陈王廷, 1597–1664) shortly after the Ming dynasty was defeated and replaced by the Qing dynasty (1644–1912). According to historical writings, after retiring from his military post to his native Chen village in Henan province, Mr. Chen spent many years synthesizing ancient philosophy with his training in internal martial arts. Under this influence, Chen-style Tai Chi Chuan (陈式太极拳) movements reflect their martial-arts origins.

Chen-style Tai Chi Chuan is known for its graceful movements and dynamic, flowing energy. Fast and explosive movements are seamlessly integrated with slow, spiraling, and coiling movements that are like undulating silk. The fast and explosive movements, such as jumping, quick kicking, and fist-striking movements, make the practice physically dynamic and engaged.

Owing to its cultural and social context, Chen-style Tai Chi Chuan was confined to a small group of individuals within a specific geographic area. As it later spread, individual martial artists modified the practice and created various styles based on their background, training, and interpretation of internal martial-arts principles. In addition to the Chen style, the five commonly recognized Tai Chi Chuan styles are the Yang (middle nineteenth century), Wu/Hao (middle to late nineteenth century), Sun (late nineteenth to early twentieth century), and Wu (late nineteenth to early twentieth century). Their distinctive characteristics are explored more deeply next.

Yang Style

Yang-style Tai Chi Chuan was developed by Luchan Yang（杨露禅, 1799–1872), a Chen-style Tai Chi Chuan student who modified the practice with a consistently slow pace; gentle, open, and flowing movements; and a focus on smooth and graceful transitions. In addition, the Yang style generally uses more upright stances, making it suitable and attractive to a broader demographic. Today, Yang-style Tai Chi Chuan is the world's most practiced form of Tai Chi Chuan.

Wu/Hao Style

Wu/Hao-style Tai Chi Chuan was developed by Yuxiang Wu (武禹襄, 1812–80), who became a Tai Chi Chuan scholar in his later years. He studied Yang-style Tai Chi Chuan with Luchan Yang and later studied Chen-style Tai Chi Chuan with Qingping Chen, a master of the Chen style. He combined these two styles into his own, which he called Wu/Hao-style Tai Chi Chuan. The Wu/Hao style uses a higher stance but smaller and more compact movements. The practice focuses on cultivating internal energy to drive the body movement.

Sun Style

This style was developed by Lutang Sun (孙禄堂, 1860–1933), a well-known internal martial-arts master. As an accomplished neo-Confucian and Daoist scholar, Mr. Sun contributed significantly to developing the theory of internal martial arts, synthesizing the concept developed by the philosophy of Daoism and the *I Ching*. Sun-style Tai Chi Chuan movements incorporate traditional Tai Chi Chuan principles with movements from Xingyi Chuan, Bagua Zhang, and several other forms of internal martial arts. The practice uses a high, upright stance and emphasizes agile footwork and small but unique stepping patterns. This form has become very popular among individuals with knee injuries and arthritis.

Wu Style

This latest style of Tai Chi Chuan was created by Jianquan Wu (吴鉴泉, 1870–1942), a Chinese martial artist and Tai Chi Chuan master. After mastering Yang-style Tai Chi Chuan, he modified the movements and created Wu-style Tai Chi Chuan, which uses a medium stance and smaller postures than those in the Yang style. It encourages practitioners to lean the body forward and backward to create extension rather than remaining centered, as in other forms of Tai Chi Chuan.

Each Tai Chi Chuan style offers a unique way for all practitioners, whatever their level of ability, to empower their physical condition and improve their mental well-being. The different ways of engaging the body in each of the styles reflects the unique interpretation of the classic texts, the principles of internal martial arts, the body's abilities, and the practice experience of the founders. The ongoing popularity of these styles shows that by empowering the mind, bodies of all abilities can be transformed. With Tai Chi Chuan, anyone can learn to use four ounces of their own power to overcome one thousand pounds of another force.

My journey of learning Tai Chi Chuan started in my late teens. Having practiced Northern Shaolin external martial arts for nearly ten years, I was attracted to Chen-style Tai Chi Chuan for its fast-paced sequences and mixed explosive movements. My first Tai Chi teacher, the late Master Gong-wei Xu, was near seventy when I became his student. He was thin, of medium height, and had a rather quiet body. It would be very hard to know just by looking at him that this ordinary-looking gentleman possessed extraordinary martial-arts skills. Watching him practicing Chen-style Tai Chi Chuan, especially the movement called "Cannon Fist," was an enjoyable, electrifying, and exhilarating experience. Later, as I learned more about internal martial-arts ideas, I became fascinated with the Yang style for its calm, graceful, and elegant way of expressing power through harmonizing and embracing movements. Though I had the opportunity to learn other styles as well, over the years the Chen and Yang styles have remained my favorites to practice and teach.

With its focus on cultivating the mind, the early development of Tai Chi Chuan not only made it a formative fighting art but also laid the foundation for it to become a healing art for mind and body. The next chapter will discuss how social and cultural challenges transformed Tai Chi Chuan from a martial art to a healing modality in modern society.

2

From a Martial Art to a Healing Art

LIKE MANY other cultural traditions, Tai Chi Chuan evolved from a martial art to a multifaceted cultural art over a long period of time and across geographic space. From Chen-style Tai Chi Chuan's appearance in a small village in Northern China over four hundred years ago, Tai Chi Chuan has gained worldwide popularity for its health and wellness benefits and its graceful, gentle, and effortless body movements. Its purpose and practice has been shaped and reconfigured by changing social and cultural environments and conditions. Owing to rapid social and cultural changes, especially since the beginning of the twentieth century in China and elsewhere, Tai Chi Chuan has continually developed, flourished, and transformed from a martial-art form to a healing art.

All styles of Tai Chi Chuan share similarities in their outwardly graceful, calm, gentle, flowing, circular, synchronized, and paced movements. The subtly flowing body movements engaged by the mind confirm the ancient wisdom that the Dao of the natural world works seamlessly in navigating change and transforming it into energy. Tai Chi Chuan is attractive to a broad demographic who work with a variety of physical and health conditions. It's an ideal way to empower the mind and body during periods of social uncertainty and drastic changes.

TAI CHI CHUAN AS A PUBLIC-HEALTH INITIATIVE IN AN ERA OF CONFLICTS

The Qing, the last dynasty in Chinese history, finally fell in 1912 and was replaced by the Republic of China. After nearly a half century of social chaos, disunity, and humiliation since the first Opium War (1839–42), the Chinese people were exhausted physically and mentally. Faced with the challenge of rebuilding the country and regaining the confidence of the masses, many martial artists, including Tai Chi Chuan masters, united together to promote traditional martial arts, including Tai Chi Chuan, as a sport to empower the people and strengthen the national spirit. Masters of various styles of Tai Chi Chuan modified their practice movements, reorienting them to promoting health for people of all physical conditions.

Despite these promising initiatives and developments, the Japanese invasion in 1937 continuously consumed the nation's resources and attention. After the end of World War II with the defeat of Japan in 1945, a civil war continued between the Nationalists and the Communists. When the war ended in 1949, the country's enormous health problems had been aggravated by years of wars and political unrest. Almost every nutritional deficiency and infectious disease was prevalent nationwide, especially in rural areas. Having to confront these complex challenges with limited resources, traditional martial-arts and healing-arts practices, including Tai Chi Chuan, were widely promoted to combat the public health crisis and became popular.

The various styles of Tai Chi Chuan that had developed earlier were often lengthy, having many movements within a particular form. This made it challenging to promote Tai Chi Chuan practice as a public healthcare initiative to benefit the general population. In 1956 a group of well-known and respected internal martial artists and Tai Chi Chuan masters collectively developed the first standardized and simplified form of Tai Chi Chuan. Based on Yang-style Tai Chi Chuan movements, this form, also called the Twenty-Four-Posture Tai Chi Chuan, significantly shortened the number of moves in traditional Tai Chi Chuan forms, making Tai Chi Chuan practice more practical for people of all levels of martial-arts training and health conditions.

Seeing Tai Chi Chuan as an embodiment of cultural wisdom and healing power, individuals, communities, healthcare providers, hospitals, and local sports and recreation organizations all embraced this simplified Tai Chi Chuan program, and soon it became the most popular form of Tai Chi Chuan practice nationwide. During the early morning hours, large crowds gathered at every urban park, practicing Tai Chi Chuan and discussing the applications of the practice to manage life and social circumstances. This simplified Tai Chi Chuan program, along with other traditional forms of Tai Chi Chuan, provided the public with a meaningful, effective, practical, and economical tool to empower their minds, regulate their emotions, strengthen their bodies, and promote their social bonding and engagement during times of uncertainty.

Since then, many Tai Chi Chuan forms of all styles have been standardized and implemented. These standardized forms can be simple or complex, the shortest form having only eight movements and the longest form having eighty-eight movements. Some were created for general practice and others were developed for advanced martial-arts competitions. Various forms of Tai Chi Chuan are practiced daily from dawn to dusk at urban parks and public spaces by millions of people, young and old, of all genders and health conditions, as a form of healing, self-care, and recreational activity.

Supported by ample research findings that explain and validate the magnificently powerful therapeutic effects of Tai Chi practice, teachers' colleges and sports and physical-education universities throughout the country have all implemented Tai Chi Chuan as a part of the standard academic curriculum, cultivating future Tai Chi Chuan professionals and researchers. Medical schools, especially traditional Chinese medical schools, offer elective courses or supplementary training in Tai Chi as part of their curriculum. In the clinical setting, Tai Chi Chuan practice has become one of the commonly recommended and applied therapeutic and rehabilitation modalities for patients with various chronic conditions.

Tai Chi Chuan in the United States and Worldwide

The fast-growing popularity of Tai Chi Chuan practice in the United States and developed countries has been attributed to many factors, including changing patterns of mortality, the recognition of the powerful relationship between the mind and body in Western medical communities, and the realization that individual lifestyle has an important impact on one's mental and physical well-being.

Since the middle of the 1960s, improved living conditions, a cleaner environment, and medical interventions not only increased the human life span but also contributed to the significant shift from an infectious disease-based to a noncommunicative and chronic disease-based pattern of mortality. The rising prevalence of heart disease, cancer, diabetes, and mental illness not only challenged the exclusivity of the germ-based disease model popular in the late nineteenth century but also contested the notion of a "magic bullet" to cure disease and a "technological fix" determinism. The new epidemiological data that was obtained using more advanced scientific instruments demonstrated that the prevalence of these health challenges among populations tends to vary according to lifestyles and a cluster of social, economic, and environmental factors, and that the significance of biological factors is relevant only to a lesser degree.

Connecting human behavior, practices, and lifestyle with states of health and disease ignited the scientific exploration of how biology, the mind, social and environmental factors, and healthcare systems interact to impact human health and disease. While scientific and medical communities analyzed their findings, complementary traditional healing methods and self-care grew in popularity across the United States. Various mind-body healing practices and programs became popular, including acupuncture, chiropractic care, homeopathy, ayurveda, naturopathy, reiki, reflexology, aromatherapy, yoga, Tai Chi, Qi Gong, and meditation. The fast growth of traditional healing methods in the United States during the 1970s and 1980s was driven by several factors, including (1) the increase in mental distress resulting from chronic health challenges; (2) the high prevalence of mental illness in the country; (3) the increasing awareness of the benefits of holistic care, which considers the interconnectedness of the mind, body, and spirit; (4) the shift of healthcare from treatment-focused to preventive-focused to empower individuals to take an active role in their healthcare; and (5) frustration with the increasingly complex, expensive, impersonal, and ineffective nature of conventional medicine.

In 1992 the US Congress established the Office of Alternative Medicine (OAM) within the National Institutes of Health (NIH). Congress elevated OAM to the National Center for Complementary and Alternative Medicine (NCCAM) in 1999. Since then, more than four hundred research proposals exploring the clinical effects of Tai Chi Chuan practice on populations with various health conditions and needs have been supported by the NIH and NCCAM. The recognition of Tai Chi Chuan as a complementary modality by the NIH and health and medical communities in the United States and throughout the world, and confirmations of the powerful therapeutic effects of Tai Chi Chuan practice revealed by their well-designed scientific studies, not only acknowledged the power of the mind in achieving well-being but also helped transform the practice from a mind-focused healing art into an evidence-based popular complementary health modality in the United States and worldwide.

Enlightened by ancient philosophy and healing practices that placed the mind at the center of human efforts to empower the body and navigate social changes, Tai Chi Chuan originated as a form of martial arts that used a force of four ounces to deflect a force of one thousand pounds. Shaped by centuries of drastic social changes, wars, and uncertainties, Tai Chi Chuan movements have been constantly modified into a multifaceted art of empowerment and healing for the mind and body, benefiting people of all health conditions across cultural and national boundaries.

3

The Principles of Tai Chi Chuan

"There's something with these ancient arts.
They don't last for centuries for nothing."
—PETER WAYNE, *The Harvard Medical School Guide to Tai Chi:
12 Weeks to a Healthy Body, Strong Heart, and Sharp Mind*

D R. WAYNE'S reference to the "something" in Tai Chi Chuan refers to its profound way of engaging the mind to empower the body. Unlike modernity's popular social constructs, Tai Chi Chuan does not view the power of the body as tangible and quantifiable or as simply muscular strength and anatomical perfection. Instead, it understands "power" and "body" as fluid and contextual, power being the manifestation of a gentle, integrated mind and body flowing as a system. This unique approach redefines strength, turning vulnerability into a source of power for practitioners and inspiring them to unlock their full potential. It not only empowers the mind but also benefits all conditions of the body within evolving social complexities and challenges in which our mind and the body's conditions and capabilities are increasingly fragmented.

The magnificent effects of Tai Chi Chuan on the well-being of mind and body are attributed to its core principles. In this chapter we will explore the modern applications of these principles, including (1) centering, (2) simplicity, (3) the mind's command of the body's movement, (4) moving with a calm and gentle force, (5) moving with synchronization and harmony, and (6) flowing with circular motions and rounded postures. Revisiting these core principles will ground your practice and equip you for an enjoyable and empowering experience of adaptive and inclusive Tai Chi Chuan.

PRINCIPLE 1: CENTERED MIND AND BODY

Being (or becoming) mentally and physically centered is the foundation of the art of Tai Chi Chuan, regardless of style. In general, being centered is considered a powerful state that results from inner and external balance and stability. When someone is centered, we also say they are grounded, focused, and in control of their emotions and actions. Many people use a big tree or a mountain as a metaphor for being centered. In the art of Tai Chi Chuan, being centered is about cultivating the ability to engage, and it is the critical element for our maxim, a force of four ounces deflecting one thousand pounds.

Centering the Body

In Tai Chi Chuan the primary focus of body centering is the lower *dantian* (丹田), an energy center and acupuncture point three inches below the navel. According to Chinese medicine, there are three dantian, or energy centers, in the body: the upper, middle, and lower dantian. Tai Chi Chuan considers the lower dantian the most important because it is located at the body's center point (figure 3-1).

To create a dynamic centering position, Tai Chi Chuan emphasizes keeping the spine straight and lengthened without being stiff and the head straight up as if suspended from above, creating gentle stability in the neck.

Relaxation is a crucial element of Tai Chi Chuan and body centering. Relaxed muscles and joints allow energy to flow efficiently and promote body sensitivity, flowing movement, and a rooted feeling.

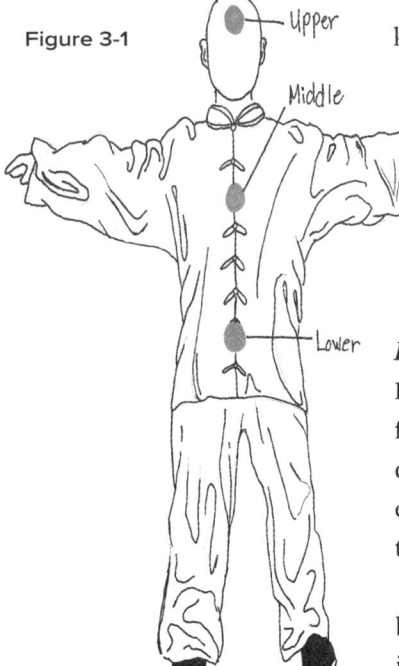

Figure 3-1

Rooting

Body centering is the foundational step for rooting. Rooting refers to the feeling of sinking the body to the ground. Imagine a tree with its roots deep in the ground. Rooting in Tai Chi Chuan allows the practitioner to effectively use the ground or a chair (if you are practicing in a seated position) to empower the flowing movements.

I often use the image of a boat sitting in the water to explain the idea of body centering and rooting in Tai Chi Chuan. When a boat sits in water, it engages the water, which creates a floating effect on the boat. In other words, to root is to rise. I use this cue, root to rise, throughout the practice instructions.

Centering the Mind

In many ancient philosophies and medical traditions, there was little distinction between the mind and the body. However, we know that the mind can move much faster than the body, and the mind and body cannot always naturally sync as one unit. In Tai Chi Chuan, a calm and engaged mind is critical for making the body able to exert a force of four ounces to deflect one thousand pounds. However, the way one uses the body can also influence the mind. This dialogue between body and mind is the foundation for the cultivation of a calm and powerful mind.

In Tai Chi Chuan a centered mind is tranquil, fluid, and engaged. This mind can become the body and can transform the body into a gentle force of unified and flowing energy. The mind is the body and the body is the mind. Without a centered mind there is no centered body, and vice versa.

So what does centering the mind mean? The answer to this seemingly simple question can be complex depending on our experience and perspective. I have answered this question in many ways but have found that one anecdote illustrates it well. One day, while making a cup of hot green tea, I noticed that all the leaves swirled and floated as in a graceful dance. But a short while later, they all gently settled at the bottom of the teacup, evoking a tranquil but dynamic state. Looking into the cup of tea, I could almost feel my mental activity settling down like the tea leaves, becoming calm and engaged with clarity and contentment.

PRINCIPLE 2: SIMPLICITY

Can you, in just one sentence , explain Tai Chi Chuan to someone who has never practiced it? That can be challenging because it requires simplicity. I have asked many new students this question throughout the years. The answers have been diverse, which reflects the multifaceted art of Tai Chi Chuan and that we interpret phenomena differently, based on our experience and perceptions. The answer that most struck me was, "Tai Chi Chuan teaches you to do a little but accomplish a lot."

Some years ago, I had one of the most enlightening conversations with Master Shu-ren Wei, an accomplished Yang-style Tai Chi Chuan master. I was still young and very fond of Chen-style Tai Chi Chuan for its dynamic movements and overt martial-arts applications. I asked the master why he picked the Yang style but not the Chen style. He responded with a question: "What has made Tai Chi Chuan the most powerful martial art?" He noticed that I was thinking too hard to answer and said with a smile, "The use of the mind." Then he asked, "Why is Tai Chi Chuan the most challenging art to master?" A few minutes later, as I tried to elaborate on my answer, he smiled and said, "The use of the mind." He continued. "Living a complex life, the mind easily and quickly becomes complicated. It will take a lot of effort to have a calm mind that has attained simplicity." He said that the essence of Tai Chi Chuan practice, regardless of the styles or forms, is about transforming structured forms into formless movements. Master Wei concluded, "In Tai Chi Chuan applications, there is no difference in styles or forms. They have only circles."

What I learned from the conversation with Master Wei is that the goal in all styles of Tai Chi Chuan is to achieve simplicity. As soon as you begin to move your body, you have already *become* Tai Chi. Simplicity or formlessness is the Dao. The ultimate skill is to do a little but accomplish a lot.

Principle 3: The Mind Commands the Body's Slow Movements

In Tai Chi Chuan practice:

1. All movements are initiated by the engagement of the mind (intentionality) through the center of one's lower back.
2. While the upper body maintains an upright position, the lower back moves gently in a circular form (leftward and rightward) to connect with and direct each body movement.
3. With a calm mind guiding the body's gentle movements, the body is held with little to no tension, and all parts of the body, especially the joints, are integrated to create the movement.

Students often ask, if most physical movements are initiated by the mind, what makes Tai Chi Chuan different from other exercises? Yes, all intentional body movements, such as walking and jogging, start with the mind. However, we can also talk to someone while walking or jogging. In Tai Chi Chuan, the moment you start to move, your mind becomes the body and the body's movements become the extension of a calm, flowing, graceful, focused, and centered mind.

Here is a story I hope further explains this principle. When I was in elementary school, one of the most anticipated and exciting events was the annual spring sporting competition at the track field. Being a part of that event was a great escape: there were no classes for two days, we could be outside, and we could bring as many snacks as we wanted. It was a holiday!

One year, toward the end of the day, a surprise event began: a 20-meter bike race among teachers. When the emcee made the announcement, all of us students were puzzled. We did not know what to think of a bike race by adults. It turned out it was not the kind of bike race we were familiar with, quite the opposite. The competition was for *last place*. Of course there were rules. The bike had to maintain forward motion and points were docked if one's foot touched the ground or if the bike crossed the track or fell. It was extraordinary. Many students were sweating as much as their teachers! My teacher was among the competitors and shared his experience with our class afterward. He told us that during the race, time seemed to slow down and everything else moved in slow motion, including his mind and the students cheering. He could feel and see every part of his body, including things he'd never felt before. He could also feel that all parts of his body were connected like a bike chain by the activated nerves in his body. He said that he'd never before felt that all the nerves were turned on like light bulbs. "That was an amazing feeling." He said that he became tense whenever he noticed there were people behind him, which made him lose his focus, connection, rhythm, and balance. He said, "Moving slowly and gracefully on a bike is far more mentally and physically exhausting than riding fast. In the end, my whole shirt was drenched."

I have told this story many times when I explain the principle that the mind commands the body's movements, and the reactions have been lovely. This principle not only defines Tai Chi but also epitomizes the concept of a force of four ounces deflecting one thousand pounds.

PRINCIPLE 4: MOVING WITH A CALM, GENTLE FORCE

This principle is an extension of the first principle. The mind is formless and can take any form. When the mind is tense, so is the body, and vice versa. Though the power of the mind is evident, the mind is complex and changes quickly. In other words, we practice Tai Chi Chuan not only when we have a sound mind or body but also to cultivate a sound mind and body. This dialectic relationship between the mind and body is a crucial contribution of Tai Chi Chuan to mental health. Many scientific studies have demonstrated the positive effect of Tai Chi Chuan practice on people with mental-health challenges. This effect is attributed to the principle of moving with a calm, gentle force, which means using pliable muscular strength while relaxing the body and sinking the body's center of gravity. Relaxing the musculature and avoiding muscle tension while moving at a slow pace not only helps to develop body sensitivity and motor control (such as balance) but also improves the circulation of energy and blood throughout the body. This creates an ideal environment for mental and physical healing.

The focus on intentionality and calm, gentle movement are defining principles of this internal martial art.

INTERNAL VS. EXTERNAL MARTIAL ARTS

I often use the following scenario to illustrate the difference between internal and external martial arts. Imagine throwing a sizable rock at a wooden object, such as a door, with full force. We all know that the rock may very well cause damage to the door. The degree of damage would depend on three factors: the quality of the rock (the hardness), the power of the throw, and the velocity of the rock. The harder the rock and the more power and speed with which you throw the rock, the more damage the rock will create. However, the result would be very different if you threw the rock with the same force and speed into a soccer net. Regardless of how hard the rock is, how much power it was thrown with, and how fast you throw it, the soccer net will not be damaged and the rock will fall gently and gracefully under the hanging soccer net. With its gentle and calming qualities, the soccer net would gently embrace the power of a thrown rock and redirect it. Therefore, in a nutshell, external martial artists primarily focus on developing their superior mental focus and physical conditions to defeat their opponents, while internal martial artists focus on developing harmonized mind and body to deflect the opponents by embracing their forces.

Principle 5: Moving with Synchronization and Harmony

One day when I was in elementary school I got into trouble by fighting with a classmate. My homeroom teacher sat me down in her office. Instead of lecturing or asking me to write a confession, she gave me a pencil. Then in a calm and angry voice, she asked me to break the pencil. I was confused and at first thought it must be a trap. When she pressed me several more times, I realized she was serious and I broke the pencil. She then opened her desk drawer and grabbed a handful of pencils. She handed them to me and asked me to break them all at once. I don't remember how many pencils there were, but it seemed like a lot. Of course I could not break them all. What was the message? We are stronger when we are aligned with others.

To cultivate a force of four ounces to deflect one thousand pounds, Tai Chi Chuan movements focus on synchronizing the energies of all body parts through gentle and circular motions to create a formless but unified energy. This energy is invisible but has a clear intention: to embrace the undesirable "invading" forces that come from outside (an opponent) or within (our own negative emotions or perceptions) and to deflect them naturally and gracefully, with harmony, like the motion of a flowing stream.

Remember the story about throwing a rock into a soccer net? Each thread used to make a soccer net may be easily broken individually, just as one pencil can be broken with a little force. However, when each thread becomes part of a soccer net, it strengthens and becomes impossible to break by a fast-moving rock, despite seeming to be soft and gentle. Likewise, the power that Tai Chi Chuan practice cultivates does not rely on the condition or ability of a specific body part but is a form of power created through the unified gentle flow of all body parts.

The soft and gentle will overcome and the stiff and rigid will be broken.

Principle 6: Flowing with Circular Motions and Rounded Postures

Circular movements and round objects are the most common phenomena in the natural world. The early Chinese philosophical treatises, including works in medicine and healing, all incorporate circular flowing motion in their models of understanding the human body and health. Cross-culturally, humans have positive associations with circular movements and round objects and have incorporated them socially and culturally, including in religious practices. In many cultures, circular movements and round objects symbolize unity, continuity, interconnectedness, harmony, flexibility, gentleness, grace, completeness, and wholeness.

Circular motion is also more natural and energy efficient than other movements and can even generate energy and create a centrifugal force. The early internal martial artists integrated this naturalistic circular motion into the martial-arts movement to achieve the effect of four ounces deflecting a thousand pounds. Flowing circular movement not only channels the opponent's force but also transforms the channeling process, empowering the deflection.

In Tai Chi Chuan practice, a movement is expressed through a circle or circles. For each circle, the first half yields to (*yin*) and channels or lures an external force toward the practitioner's body center; the second half redirects (*yang*) the external force. Placing the center of the circle at the practitioner's lower back, the flowing movement around and toward the practitioner's center not only empowers but also transforms and redirects the opponent's force.

Regarding the principle of round postures in Tai Chi Chuan movements, structural integrity is at play. Round shapes distribute forces evenly, which helps to prevent concentrated stress points. This makes round objects, like spheres and cylinders, stronger and more resistant to deformation or collapse than other shapes. A wheel can handle a lot of weight because the force is distributed evenly around it. Therefore, a mind with no edges becomes empowered and promotes the flow of energy, becoming a true force of nature.

TAI CHI AS A TREE OF MIND-BODY ENGAGEMENT

Deeply rooted in and nourished by early Chinese philosophical and cultural wisdom, these core principles of Tai Chi, serving as the trunk of the giant Tai Chi tree, have guided the development of Tai Chi Chuan for centuries. The branches of this tree, symbolized by the five styles of Tai Chi Chuan, powerfully illustrate the various ways of empowering our vulnerable bodies through mind-engaged body flow.

Inspired by the root of the Tai Chi tree, wheelchair and adaptive and inclusive Tai Chi Chuan were developed. The success of implementing the thirteen-posture wheelchair Tai Chi Chuan program at the 2008 Paralympics and the seven-posture inclusive Tai Chi Chuan program throughout the US Department of Veterans Affairs healthcare system exemplifies the adaptability and inclusivity of Tai Chi Chuan. The practice transforms disability into ability, inspiring us with its capacity to reach and empower a wider range of practitioner abilities. In the next chapter, we share practitioner stories of how this program empowered and transformed their minds and bodies.

4

Tai Chi Applications for Modern Challenges

O N SEPTEMBER 5, 2008, fifty wheelchair Tai Chi Chuan practitioners dressed in white silk uniforms and moving in slow, graceful harmony premiered the "Thirteen Postures of Wheelchair Tai Chi Chuan" on the main stage of the Paralympics Cultural Festival, one of the kickoff events for the opening ceremony of the Beijing 2008 Olympics. "They moved so beautifully, and it was so inspirational—as if they were dancing in the chair," was how one of the reporters on the scene described them.

To learn how wheelchair Tai Chi Chuan practitioners perceive the benefits of their practice, the project team conducted a structured interview with the forty-nine wheelchair practitioners who participated in the demonstration at the 2008 Paralympics. Participants from various regions of China were selected to represent their regions through a competitive selection process conducted by regional disability organizations. About half of the forty-nine practitioners were wheelchair users; the others used crutches or canes to manage their daily activities. They had all practiced wheelchair Tai Chi Chuan for at least one year, and over 80 percent reportedly practiced at least once a day for at least thirty minutes. Over 80 percent of respondents indicated that they enjoyed both group and solo practices and expressed their joy and satisfaction in the practices.

"WE CAN PERFORM IT BEAUTIFULLY"

The team asked each participant to provide a list of noticeable changes that they experienced since participating in wheelchair Tai Chi Chuan practice. The respondents reported 173 positive changes, ranging from physical improvements to enhanced social and psychological well-being. These changes, experienced by a majority of participants, serve as tangible evidence of the benefits of wheelchair Tai Chi Chuan. Of these 173 positive changes in well-being, 53 percent were physical and 47 percent were social and psychological.

- 78 percent of participants reported that the practice improved many physical ailments and enhanced their general health and quality of sleep.
- 57 percent of participants mentioned that the practice alleviated various types of body pain and improved joint conditions, including their range of motion.
- 70 percent of participants reported changes related to emotional well-being, such as becoming more cheerful, becoming more optimistic, having fewer mood swings, and being calmer.
- More remarkably, 67 percent of participants used phrases such as "became more confident about life," "improved self-confidence," and "improved self-image" to describe their experienced changes in the context of social engagement.

The project team also conducted a focus-group interview to explore why many participants experienced a positive change in self-confidence through the practice. When asked why so many people felt that participating in wheelchair Tai Chi Chuan had improved their self-confidence, some shared that the enhanced physical and emotional conditions through the practice gave them great confidence in managing their family and social lives. Many also said that they were encouraged to practice wheelchair Tai Chi Chuan in public places since the practice does not highlight their disabilities and gives them a sense of normalcy (Tai Chi Chuan is a widespread fitness practice in public spaces). A male participant commented: "When we practice at the park every morning, people look at us with admiration, and it makes me feel so proud and confident. Now I always look forward to going out to practice wheelchair Tai Chi Chuan." When asked why practicing at the park was so important, a female participant added: "That is where [able-bodied] people practice Tai Chi Chuan in the morning, and we wanted to show them that we [people with disabilities] can also perform Tai Chi Chuan, and we can perform it beautifully." Another male participant shared this story with the group: As his health deteriorated, he became wheelchair-bound. His depression worsened when he learned that his teenage son had become very quiet in school. One day, shortly after he had started to practice Tai

Chi Chuan, his son told him that many of his friends wanted to come to the house and watch him practice. His son was excited to see his father practicing wheelchair Tai Chi Chuan and told his school friends that his father was a wheelchair martial artist. "Practicing wheelchair Tai Chi Chuan not only changed me but also changed how my son sees me," the man said with a smile.

During the conversation, a participant said he felt like a bird while practicing wheelchair Tai Chi Chuan: "It would be hard for people who do not use a wheelchair to imagine how we [wheelchair users] perceive space. Before making every move, I must calculate how far I can go. My physical and mental spaces are determined by how far and high I can reach. The circular movement of Tai Chi Chuan changed my mental image of my physical boundary. I can move gracefully and infinitely when I am practicing wheelchair Tai Chi Chuan, which makes me feel like I am so free."

Toward the end of the conversation, many participants expressed their heartfelt appreciation for the opportunity to be part of a historical event—demonstrating wheelchair Tai Chi Chuan at the Thirteenth Paralympics. One participant explained,

> People like me had never dreamed that we could one day be invited to demonstrate our ability and have our "disabled body" appreciated on an international stage. I had always been depressed about my disability since I was a young girl. I was always concerned about how others would look at me, and I often perceived myself as a burden to my family and society because of my disability. Being selected to participate in the wheelchair Tai Chi Chuan demonstration for the Paralympics was the greatest gift of my life. It tells people like me that we are not a burden and can contribute to society and the world just like others.

Her emotional words immediately met with loud applause from everyone in the room. Many participants tried to help one another hold their crutches to stand up, showing their support for the shared sentiment of ability. I noticed that several participants had tears in their eyes.

Rising from Stillness: Working with People with Spinal Cord Injury

Since its debut at the 2008 Paralympics, the broader applications and creative implications of the wheelchair Tai Chi Chuan program as either an intervention or self-care modality have been recognized worldwide. In 2008 I led a team of researchers who partnered with the Siskin Physical Rehabilitation Hospital of Chattanooga to conduct a pilot study on the effectiveness of wheelchair Tai Chi Chuan practice to promote physical-fitness participation for people with severe ambulatory challenges due to spinal cord injury or disorder (SCI/D). Considering their physical conditions and their psychological and social needs, a short four-movement adaptive wheelchair Tai Chi Chuan program was developed to provide participants with a therapeutic, enjoyable, and transformative experience that did not highlight their disabilities.

Participants had various degrees of limitation, from needing to use a cane to needing a motorized wheelchair. Some had spinal cord injuries and others had suffered strokes or had multiple sclerosis, Parkinson's disease, or a host of conditions in between. They participated in a 45-minute group practice session twice weekly. Participants were also encouraged to practice daily at home following an instructional DVD provided by the project team. They were asked to maintain a daily written log on their home practice. A student-researcher on the project team called each participant daily to answer questions about their home practice. Throughout this eight-week exploratory study, many participants reported a number of positive effects:

- Daily activities no longer caused pain.
- There was a greater ability to maneuver, such as transferring from chair to car with much more ease.
- There was improvement in balance and flexibility.
- There was better blood circulation.
- There was increased movement or mobility after a stroke, and the practice had a positive impact on their outlook on themselves and their lives.
- Several participants shared with the group that watching themselves and others move gracefully without feeling "disabled" gave them a sense of hope and normality.

At the end of the study, participants demanded to continue the wheelchair Tai Chi Chuan class. Encouraged by the participants' enthusiasm, Dr. William Johnson, the instructor, agreed to continue the practice sessions. The eight-week study turned into an eight-year practice. During the eight years, many new participants joined the class. At the end of the eighth year, Dr. Johnson had to step down as the instructor for the group owing to his busy clinical practice. The class continued for a few more years, led by Ms. R., one of the original participants in the study and later certified as a wheelchair Tai Chi Chuan instructor.

TO FLOW IS TO TRANSFORM

One of the instructional strategies we used in this project that was enthusiastically embraced by participants was the repetitive practice through following along, a movement-guided practice that allows participants to repeat a movement or set of movements by following the instructor. This method can be combined with guided practice through narrative and music to achieve specific effects. For example, when an instructor finishes teaching a movement or movements, she asks participants to follow along with her as they practice the movements five times consecutively. In each repetition, the instructor guides the practice by focusing on a specific objective and area of importance, including (1) body posture, (2) the synchronization of the movement and breathing, (3) mind-engaged body flow, (4) nature- or movement-oriented figurative language to connect the mental image, and (5) body movements to transform the physical condition and empower the mind and body flow. For the last round, the instructor might have the participants follow along with background music without any instructions.

> Music is used to accompany practice and create a calm and meditative atmosphere. It enhances mental focus and body relaxation during practice. Rhythmic music can also help with timing movements and the breath, promoting a constructive and harmonious flow of the mind and body.

This method was developed by working with Tai Chi students who enjoyed practicing just a few favorite movements rather than the long form. Many people told me that repeatedly practicing a single movement or a few movements helped them understand the movement and allowed them to synergize the flow of mind, body, and breath more quickly.

Considering the physical, psychological, and life circumstances of the participants, the team felt this method would be especially suitable for the project's objectives and targeted population. Using a short form with four movements (and making each movement a practice unit) had many benefits: it eased participants' worries about remembering multiple movements, more effectively helped to build participants' self-confidence, and provided the benefits of Tai Chi Chuan practice within a short period. Thus, it was more likely to promote participants' intrinsic motivation to practice. The instructions for practicing individual movement are detailed in the last chapter of this book.

ADAPTIVE TAI CHI FOR PEOPLE WHO ENDURE SEVERE MENTAL ILLNESS

Many people have disabilities that prevent them from engaging in conventional physical activities. In a program at a residential home for adults with severe mental illness, we modified the short four-movement form, making it suitable for practice while standing or sitting in a wheelchair. One of our strategies was to have participants start the practice in the sitting position and progress to the standing position if they could. Realizing that many residents were also challenged by an inability to mentally focus, we decided to incorporate a few adaptations: repetitive practice through following along, guided practice with instructions, and practice with music. These creative changes provided the participants with a calming experience of mental and physical flow that included breathing and a healing connection to nature by listening to music with nature sounds. This approach was designed to promote a new confidence in empowering the mind and body. Led by two Tai Chi practitioners trained to work with severely mentally ill individuals, each residential home held a 40-minute Tai Chi practice session twice weekly. The two instructors, one sitting in a chair and the other standing, performed the four-posture adaptive Tai Chi Chuan movements to calming, soothing music with nature sounds. Many participants watched the performance with joy and intrigued facial expressions. We asked each resident how they felt while watching the performance, and while their replies were varied, they all used the words "beautiful," "flowing," "calming," "relaxing," and "water." One said, "It almost put me to sleep."

Based on their enthusiastic responses, we engaged the residents in a lively conversation about making our minds and bodies beautiful, calming, and flowing, like water and clouds. These discussions established a fantastic platform to launch a Tai Chi Chuan program that, from the participants' perspective, created mental and physical beauty and flow through physical exercise and music with nature sounds.

Working with Inner-City Youth

Many inner-city youths face innumerable daunting health risks. Broken families, widespread street violence, poor economic conditions, and lack of resources and care structures contribute to the rise of many health problems and behavioral and emotional challenges. "Many learned to use anger to deal with emotional problems," a veteran youth counselor of the Boys & Girls Club shared. Developing effective, suitable, and sustainable intervention programs that could effectively alter the current trend is imperative but challenging.

With the support of the US Health Resource and Service Administration, we collaborated with the Boys & Girls Club in a metropolitan area of the southeastern United States to introduce a short, adaptive Tai Chi Chuan program to a group of inner-city youths who attended the summer camp hosted by the organization. One of the aims of this project was to explore how Tai Chi practice could influence participants' perceptions of power. Twenty-five youths—fourteen girls and eleven boys aged seven to fourteen—participated in a 30-minute session once a week for eight weeks.

Considering the age range of this group, we created a four-movement Tai Chi Chuan form in which two movements were from the Yang style and two from the Chen style. By mixing the graceful, slow, and flowing Yang-style movements with the fast and dynamically expressed energy of the Chen-style movements, we intended to give the participants an embodied experience of unified power through gentle flow while they enjoyed a simple but fun and engaging introduction to the art of Tai Chi Chuan.

Taking the truism "a picture is worth a thousand words" to heart, the program instruction focused on using natural metaphors and similes to guide learning and practicing the four Tai Chi movements to clarify the complex ideas, such as stand like a tree, yield like a bamboo, flow like a river.

Shortly after the eight-week Tai Chi practice ended, a program evaluation team conducted two focus-group interviews with a group of four girls and a group of six boys. The team asked each group what they most remembered from participating in the classes.

Girls Group	Boys Group
1. Yield and redirect	1. Yield and redirect
2. To root is to maintain one's balance	2. Gentle with balance
3. Calm but focused	3. Focus
4. Gentle but with direction	4. Still and gentle
5. Yield like bamboo, redirect like a wave	5. Flexible like bamboo
6. Stand like a tree	6. Stand like a tree
7. Flow like water	7. Flow like water
8. Golden rooster (stand on one leg)	8. Golden rooster (stand on one leg)
9. Sit like a mountain	9. Look through the wall
10. Walk like a cat	10. Push the mountain
11. Punch like a whip	11. Move like the wind
	12. Still
	13. Deflect distractions

The participants were then asked to identify the top three phrases they thought were important for their everyday lives. For the girls' group, "flow like water" was selected by everyone, "yield and redirect" was selected by three girls, and "punch like a whip" and "yield like bamboo" each received two votes. When the evaluation team asked why they thought "flow like water" was the most important metaphor for everyday life, all four girls agreed that it helped them stay calm throughout the day whenever they got stressed.

For the boys' group, "deflect distractions" received six votes and "focus" and "golden rooster" each got five votes. Both "deflect distractions" and "focus" had real-life applications in avoiding violence, focusing on school and home responsibilities, and having courage.

A few years ago, as I walked across my university campus, a student stopped me and asked with a delightful smile, "You are Dr. Guo, right? Do you remember me?" I found his face familiar, but I couldn't pinpoint where we had met or when. "Stand like a tree!" he said, his voice filled with excitement and pride. Yes, he was one of the young people who participated in the Tai Chi Chuan classes I led five years previously. He was now a student majoring in social work. After that encounter, I often wish there were a way of knowing how those young people are doing.

A Seven Years' Journey: Working with Veterans with Disabilities

Based on the positive feedback from vulnerable populations both in the United States and abroad, and partnering with Dr. William Johnson, we collaborated with the Division of Physical Medicine and Rehabilitation Service in a Veterans Affairs medical center in the southeast United States to explore the feasibility of applying the wheelchair Tai Chi Chuan program to promote fitness for veterans with ambulatory limitations due to injury. We started with six months of "fieldwork" at the VA medical center, where we provided several wheelchair classes for veterans with disabilities and introduction training to healthcare providers. We learned that in order to develop and implement an effective and sustainable program, the design and implementation strategies had to be context specific.

Veterans with disabilities have diverse physical conditions. The one-size-fits-all or standard approach would be less effective and would discourage practice, since one practice method may suit some but not others. A sustainable practice modality has to apply the principles of Tai Chi Chuan effectively and, at the same time, has to highlight participants' abilities in order to be empowering.

Veterans with disabilities, including post-traumatic stress disorder (PTSD), face unique challenges in managing their health and their emotional lives. Healthcare providers can best understand these challenges (many are veterans themselves) and can best modify specific Tai Chi Chuan movements that were initially developed for the veteran ambulatory population according to their body conditions and health needs.

Inclusive Tai Chi Chuan

During the six months of fieldwork at the VA medical center, many healthcare providers said that they enjoyed learning and practicing the thirteen-posture wheelchair series, but they thought that the form was too long and would be challenging to teach to veterans. Therapeutic programs in many VA medical centers are usually just a few weeks long, though duration can vary slightly.

I also learned that the concept of "ambulatory disability" is fluid within the veteran population. Not everyone who has an ambulatory disability uses an assistive device, and not everyone who is without an ambulatory disability can participate in meaningful physical activities. Many healthcare providers said that the biggest challenge is identifying a program that everyone can do together without indirectly creating a feeling of exclusivity among veteran participants.

With invaluable feedback from healthcare providers and veterans with disabilities and their family members, I modified the thirteen-posture wheelchair Tai Chi Chuan program and developed an inclusive seven-posture version. Focusing on "yielding and redirecting" through gentle and flowing movements in conjunction with deep breathing, this innovative program offers five different practice modalities, including walking, seated, standing, wheelchair, and individual. It has several key benefits:

1. It can be practiced by participants with different body conditions in a group setting.
2. Participants who use the four practice modalities (seated, standing, walking, and in a wheelchair) in a group-practice setting can easily synchronize their movements while moving together in unison.
3. It offers a model of transitional learning and practice. For example, participants with knee or lower-back injuries can start the practice seated, in which position they can comfortably rotate the spine without overloading the sacroiliac joints. Since all stress on body joints is minimized, there is no fear that the movements might cause pain or injury. Once the participants gain confidence in the upper body movements, it will be easier to transition to the standing and walking practice modalities.
4. The wheelchair, seated, standing, and walking modalities can also be used as a therapeutic and rehabilitative progression model.
5. Finally, the program can promote family practice. Many veterans who participated in the wheelchair Tai Chi classes in the medical center were accompanied by their spouses. Knowing that the veterans enjoyed the practice so much made their spouses want to practice with them at home.

Inclusivity has always been central to the art of Tai Chi Chuan, which emphasizes mind over body, not physical or tangible power, and regards power as contextual, fluid, and a function of mind-engaged body flow. Therefore, each practice modality in inclusive Tai Chi Chuan demonstrates that every body condition offers a unique platform for cultivating physical, emotional, and social well-being.

Many veteran participants and healthcare providers have embraced this inclusive approach. They told us that it changed their perception of their "inability" and gave them a progressive trajectory. Veterans commented things like, "I was so excited when I was told that a Tai Chi program was developed for people like me," and "Sitting in a chair, flowing with gentle martial-arts moves alongside my fellow veterans, is the only time I do not feel disabled." Another shared,

> I started doing it in a wheelchair. Since then, I have stood up and I am doing it standing. When I make my turns, I have to take baby steps to keep my balance, but because of the program and all the camaraderie, I am not doing it in a wheelchair. I use a walker . . . This program is giving me two things every day: I can see another sunset and I can see another sunrise.

And another veteran said,

> The inclusive Tai Chuan program has benefited me greatly over the years. I can use the four different modalities (sitting, standing, walking, and wheelchair) during different seasons of my life. I was able to do the program sitting after having two major surgeries and recovering. I could do the program standing and sitting most days. The standing program also helped me with postsurgery physical therapy to strengthen my balance and posture and regain muscle strength . . . I am currently in postoperative physical therapy and my surgeons and physical therapists are amazed at how fast I have progressed after having foot reconstructive surgery a few months ago.

Healthcare providers also found that the inclusive approach significantly benefited the participants physically and mentally. One of them explained: "For example, with back pain, it is important to understand what positions may increase pain and for what duration. If maintaining one position for a long time increases pain, it is important to be able to alternate. Everyone has different needs, and therefore it is important to be able to modify the positioning as needed."

Partnering with Healthcare Providers

Our many interviews with healthcare providers provided great insight into the benefits of developing partnerships with VA healthcare providers in the program-delivery process. In addition to the advantages previously discussed, the benefits of training VA healthcare providers include the following:

1. Healthcare providers are a vulnerable population. Many healthcare providers within the VA healthcare system are veterans themselves. Practice can provide them with an embodied experience of the benefits of Tai Chi Chuan, contributing to their mental and physical well-being. A healthcare provider who completed the training shared, "I have found a remedy for myself."
2. Having experienced the benefits of Tai Chi Chuan practice, they could be more encouraging and effective in applying the program in their clinical practice.
3. As in many other body-movement interventions, the instructors' ability to embody the flowing beauty and the spirit of Tai Chi Chuan is a powerful way to inspire others to learn. Growing up in a martial-arts culture taught me that teachers are differentiated by skill and ability. My favorite quote is: "The ordinary teacher tells. The good teacher explains. The great teacher embodies."

A VA healthcare provider who completed the instructional training said,

> Observing an instructor or healthcare provider performing Tai Chi movements can capture the interest of veterans with disabilities and inspire them. Some of these veterans may have a preconceived notion that Tai Chi is a practice for old people or the physically weak. Others may believe they cannot do the movements because they have some disability or limitations. By watching someone else perform the movements, especially when the demonstrator has adapted them to the ability level of

the audience and demonstrates their martial-arts applications, veterans can see that Tai Chi is accessible to them and they can benefit from the practice.

Another VA healthcare provider and instructor commented:

> The ability to perform Tai Chi Chuan as a healthcare instructor demonstrates a commitment to the well-being and holistic care of veterans with disabilities. It signals an understanding of their unique challenges and a willingness to provide tailored solutions. This level of expertise and dedication can significantly enhance the interest and participation of veterans with disabilities, as they are more likely to feel valued, respected, and supported in their Tai Chi Chuan journey.

In 2021 we conducted a national survey among healthcare providers who provided the inclusive Tai Chi Chuan program to veterans with various physical and health conditions and needs. All survey participants reported modifying the movements to meet their participants' needs. One healthcare provider wrote,

> Healthcare professionals and instructors proficient in Tai Chi Chuan can provide specialized guidance and support to disabled veterans. They possess the expertise to modify and adapt the movements and techniques to suit individual abilities and limitations. This tailored approach ensures that participants feel safe, comfortable, and empowered to engage in the practice, knowing their needs are understood and addressed. By providing appropriate modifications, instructors can make Tai Chi Chuan accessible to a broader range of individuals, including those with mobility limitations, chronic pain, or other disabilities.

The Instructional Training

Providing instructional training to VA healthcare providers is the core component of the endeavor to make the inclusive Tai Chi Chuan program benefit a broad population of healthcare providers and veterans, including those with disabilities.

Since the primary population that this inclusive program focuses on includes individuals with physical and psychological challenges, the pedagogical considerations differ from those that teach Tai Chi Chuan as a form of martial arts—that is, as a sport or a fitness practice for the general population. In addition to the emphasis on cultivating health-care providers' and participants' efficiency in Tai Chi Chuan movements and practices, and the ability to modify the movements according to the individual participant's physical ability and psychological condition, the pedagogical method also focuses the mind to empower the body using (1) language suggestive of martial arts and (2) nature metaphors to guide veteran practitioners through the movements.

1. Martial-Arts Applications

Most veterans we worked with during the six-month fieldwork at the VA medical center shared their fondness for the martial-arts aspect of Tai Chi Chuan movements. Recognizing that Tai Chi Chuan practice could empower participants and renew their sense of self-confidence and resilience despite their disabilities, the program focused on providing participants with the martial-arts implications of each movement by using its narrative of "yielding and embracing" and "redirecting and transforming" as the participants flowed from one circle to the next.

Although many healthcare providers are not experienced martial-arts practitioners, they were equally enthusiastic about the martial-arts applications of Tai Chi Chuan movements. They told us that showing them makes the learning and practice more appealing, as many veterans often have difficulty visualizing the benefit of the slower movements. One healthcare provider shared,

> Though I do not have a martial arts background, I know that many veterans I work with do. Even if they had not participated in formal martial-arts practice, all of them acquired combat and self-defense skills at some point during their military training. Often, when an individual experiences an injury or disease that causes disability, they are also left with a sense of vulnerability. Just as martial-arts and combat training instill survival and self-defense skills, inclusive Tai Chi Chuan can restore a sense of strength and counteract the vulnerability that an individual with a disability may be experiencing.

2. The Use of Nature Metaphors

The use of nature-oriented metaphors to describe movements has been the general tradition for many martial arts, particularly Tai Chi Chuan, whose development was inspired and shaped by ancient wisdom and the human admiration of nature. Not only do many Tai Chi Chuan movements imitate the way of the natural world, but their names are also associated with powerful, graceful animals and natural objects. Therefore, since its inception, Tai Chi Chuan has been both a practice and a metaphor for the way of the natural world. Such features were intended to validate the ancient wisdom that humans are a part of the natural world. They are an effective way of communicating complex constructs, such as mind-engaged body centering, through familiar imagery, such as "the golden rooster stands on one leg."

Therefore, using nature metaphors and naturalistic movements to guide participants through physical and emotional stress is a practical way of cultivating mental and physical empowerment. For example, while leading a group of seated Tai Chi Chuan practitioners, the instruction to "sit like a mountain, flow like a river" not only allows the participants to view their physical condition in a natural context but also provides an embodied experience of harmony and empowerment within the complexity and challenging aspects of life, regardless of the health condition.

Healthcare providers and instructors often shared the positive feedback they received from their veteran participants. When they repeatedly used these nature metaphors and analogies to communicate the ideas and principles of the movements, it allowed the participants' minds to calmly and naturally connect with familiar natural objects and their body movements to flow as if there were no disability. It also made their body movements purposeful, as if, for example, they were overcoming negative emotions through yielding and redirecting like bamboo.

The inclusive Tai Chi Chuan program to benefit veterans with disabilities in partnership with VA healthcare providers was overwhelmingly well received for its effectiveness in promoting the physical and mental well-being of veterans with disabilities during the early model testing period. A program director at a Georgia VA medical center stated,

The adaptive Tai Chi program has profoundly impacted the veterans we serve and provide therapy to within the VA. The seven forms are highly adaptable to the functional level of the participant and provide a great platform for improving Tai Chi skills within the seven forms. Currently we have veterans within inpatient and out-patient populations and via telehealth who participate in the seven forms that a handful of clinicians teach at my VA medical center. Veterans report enjoying this practice and feeling better both emotionally and physically through this practice.

The director of the PTSD unit at a Louisiana VA medical center said,

This training will allow us to greatly expand our Tai Chi offerings to veterans throughout our facility, including several community-based outpatient clinics that provide care to our rural and traditionally underserved populations. This training significantly increases our ability to provide this incredibly beneficial practice to Veterans across our system and has also energized our staff.

As word spread throughout the US Veterans Affairs healthcare system, many VA medical centers requested that their healthcare providers be trained in this program. From 2017 to 2023, funded with seven consecutive years of grants by the US Department of Veterans Affairs, the project team, partnering with adaptive Tai Chi international instructors, conducted 107 instructional training courses of the inclusive Tai Chi Chuan for veterans program for 1,480 healthcare providers of eighty VA medical centers in forty-six states, including Puerto Rico. According to data from a VA medical center in Tennessee, the healthcare providers who participated in the training during 2022–23 alone implemented the inclusive Tai Chi Chuan program to 3,594 veterans with disabilities.

In part 2, I provide step-by-step instructions and illustrations of each of the five practice modalities of this inclusive and adaptive Tai Chi Chuan program.

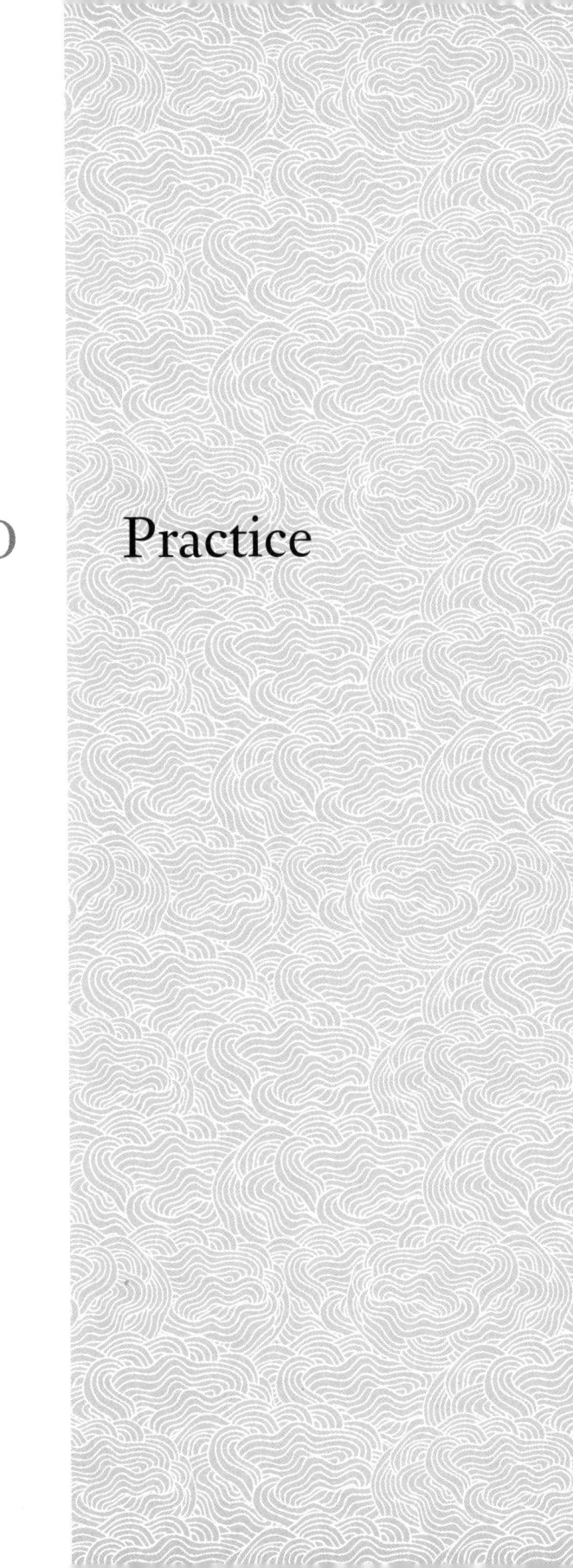

PART TWO   Practice

5

Sit Like a Mountain and Move Like a Wheel
Wheelchair Tai Chi Chuan

THE SIMILE "sit like a mountain and move like a wheel" restores the body in the wheelchair to its rightful place in the natural world. Throughout this book, such similes and metaphors remind the differently abled of their ability and power. The mental image of a giant mountain inspires awe and is humbling, and the movement of wheels can be calming, mesmerizing, and like overcoming obstacles. The similes focus the mind to empower the body's movements, a mere four ounces moving one thousand pounds.

The instructions and illustrations in this chapter provide valuable references to anyone curious about learning the ideas and methods of this therapeutic, transformative, and empowering modality. That said, it would be challenging to master the art if you have no prior Tai Chi Chuan experience and do not have a teacher.

First, a few points to help you understand and use this program.

The benefits of this modality: I have seen many people, all with different body conditions, benefit from the practice. Many are ambulatory but because of injuries have difficulty engaging in conventional physical activities without experiencing body pain. "This is the only sports activity that makes me forget my disability when I do it," said one participant with multiple disabilities.

The key feature: The central idea of this modality is to make the wheelchair motion a part of the seated movements. When we turn and push the wheels, we need to make the wheelchair motion a part of body flow. This takes practice.

Space or location for practice: The space required for practicing wheelchair Tai Chi Chuan is minimal, about 10 x 6 feet. Any area that is wheelchair friendly, has a smooth, hard floor, and is barrier-free will work.

The wheelchair: Any wheelchair with a straight back post and removable armrests will support this practice. Since one must move and turn the wheelchair, a wheelchair with footrests will provide a safer and steadier experience.

The body: The wheelchair practice focuses on integrating body, breath, chair, and movements into one dynamic flow of energy or force. For an optimal experience, be sure that your lower back is pressed firmly against the back of the chair and keep an upright posture throughout the practice. Many people also find that placing a rolled-up towel behind the lower back improves their support and makes the chair movements easier and more comfortable.

The 45-degree rotating requirement: The instruction to rotate and turn the body 45 degrees left or right serves as a reference point; the degree of the turn will depend on the body's condition and other factors. I also emphasize the importance of initiating each movement through the torso or the lower back. Gentle, circular, and a wide range of turning movements during the practice reinforces the mind and body connection, promotes circulation and the lower back's range of motion, and enhances the experience of empowerment.

Disclaimer: Engaging in any physical exercise can lead to discomfort or injury. These practices are not intended as medical advice or treatment and they do not replace medical supervision and treatment. Please consult with your primary healthcare provider before starting the practice.

⁞ Preparatory Posture (Figure 5-1)

While sitting, keep the head, neck, and body upright, holding the head straight up as if suspended from above by a thread. The eyes look straight ahead, their gaze like two swords that look through everything in front of you. Press the body against the back of the chair and keep the shoulders relaxed and down. Release all tension from the arms and allow them to hang gently from your sides (figure 5-1).

Helpful pointers: To sit is to rise: When in a sitting position, imagine you are sitting like a boat in the water. As your body and mind sink downward, the water (chair) raises your body up.

Unite the body, mind, breath, and chair: Sit vertically and have your back pressing against the back of the chair.

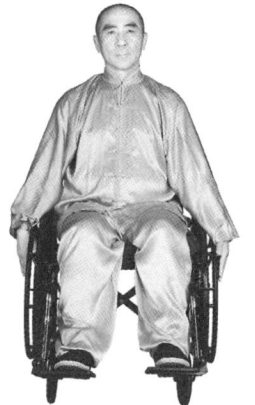

Figure 5-1

⠿ Commencement (Figures 5-2 to 5-4)

Slowly lift both arms to shoulder height, palms facing down, with elbows bent and wrists relaxed (figure 5-2).

In one continuous movement, bring the arms forward, shoulder-width apart and shoulder height, with elbows pointing down and palms relaxed and facing down (figure 5-3).

Slowly bend and drop the elbows and draw the arms slightly inward. Press the forearms downward until the palms are a few inches above your knees (figure 5-4).

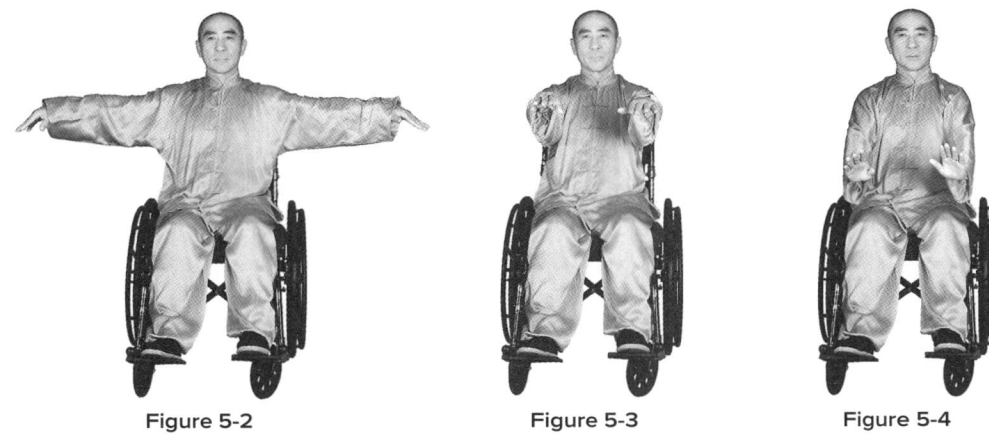

| Figure 5-2 | Figure 5-3 | Figure 5-4 |

Helpful pointers: To sit is to rise: As the arms slowly rise to shoulder height, keep the elbows slightly bent and pointed down. Imagine the force lifting your arms comes from the torso as your body sinks downward.

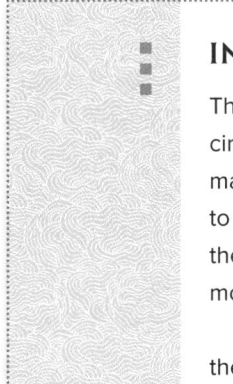

INSIGHTS

The commencement is a two-part circular movement. The first part of the circle (figures 5-1 to 5-3) denotes the energy of yielding or gathering the massive incoming forces (or stressors) together and bringing them close to your center; the second part of the circle (figures 5-3 to 5-4) denotes the energy of redirecting the compiled force downward through a flowing movement. As you push both arms down, feel your body rise.

Many people like to visualize the sun rising when raising their arms and the sun setting when pressing their arms down.

Push without pushing: When pressing your arms downward, focus on the center of the palms. Imagine you are slowly pushing a beach ball into the water.

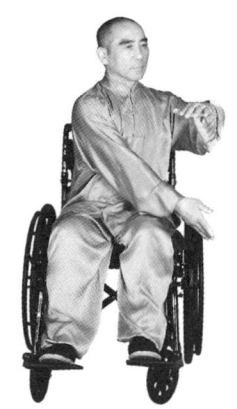

Figure 5-5

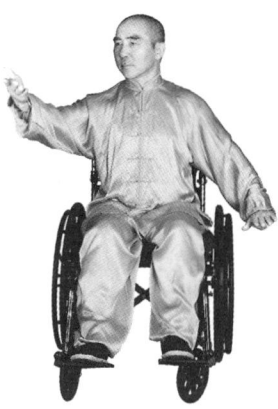

Figure 5-6

: Movement 1: Parting the Wild Horse's Mane (Figures 5-4 to 5-6)

From the position in figure 5-4, slowly rotate the torso 45 degrees to the left, then open both arms slightly before circling the left arm to chest height and sweeping the right hand with palm facing left over your knees to the left, as though you are holding a big ball under the left arm (figure 5-5).

Next, rotate the torso 45 degrees to the right, and slowly press the left palm down toward the back and stop at the left hip, outside the wheel. Synchronize the turning, raising the right hand to the chest height before swinging it out 45 degrees to the right, with the palm facing up and ending at a position just slightly below eye level (figure 5-6).

Helpful pointers: When taking the "hold a ball" position (figure 5-5), keep the left palm at shoulder height and drop the elbow that is pointing down; look to the left.

Rotating the torso and swinging the right hand to the right is similar to throwing a frisbee from low left upward to the right to eye height. Let the body's rotation lead the arm's movements.

Always remain centered. When you are in the motion illustrated in figures 5-5 and 5-6, be sure that your body is upright and keep the body center from leaning forward or sideways.

: INSIGHTS

The first half of the circle for this movement (figures 5-4 to 5-5) denotes the energy of yielding to an incoming force. The "holding the ball" position builds energy through the yielding motion. When holding the ball to the left, the torso should be slightly folded inward, and the low-back area should feel like a gently pressed spring ready to open to the right. The second part of the circle (figures 5-5 to 5-6) denotes the energy (built from holding the ball) of redirecting the incoming force through an outwardly flowing movement.

⁞ Movement 2: Brush Knee and Push Hand (Figures 5-6 to 5-9)

From figure 5-6, as you rotate the torso slightly to the right, slide your right hand down to the side with the palm facing up. At the same time, float the left arm up to the left side of the forehead (figure 5-7).

The right hand, with the palm facing up, swings out and up with a circle to the side of the right ear, turning the palm to face forward and dropping the elbow. The left arm crosses in front of the face, passing the right shoulder to the front of the right hip (figure 5-8).

As you rotate the torso 45 degrees to the left, sweep the left hand down and outward across the front of the knees to the outside of the left wheel with the palm facing down. At the same time, press the right hand toward the left at 45 degrees, with the palm facing forward and at nose height (figure 5-9).

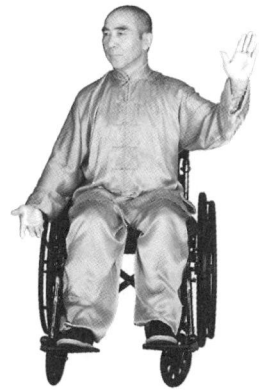
Figure 5-7

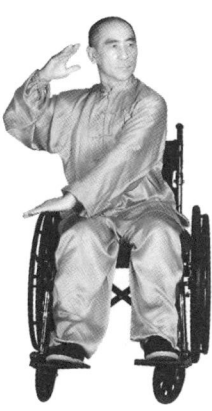
Figure 5-8

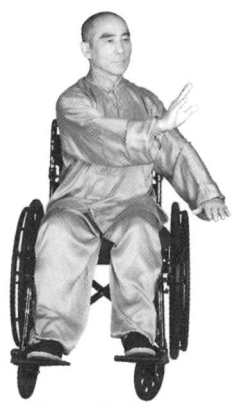
Figure 5-9

Helpful pointers: The chair is the source of power. When pushing your right palm forward (45 degrees to the left), make sure that the power of pushing comes from the weight of your body and pressing your back against the chair.

Always keep the body centered. When pushing, be sure that the body is upright and avoid having

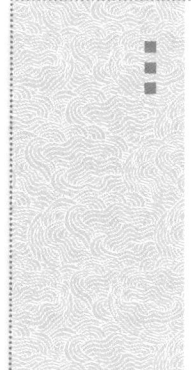

⁞ APPLICATION

The first half of the circle for this movement (figures 5-6 to 5-8) denotes the energy of yielding or rendering an incoming force. The second part of the circle (figures 5-8 to 5-9) denotes the energy of redirecting the incoming force through an outwardly flowing movement of the body and arms.

the body lean forward or sideward. Press the body slightly against the back of the chair.

⁞ Transitional Movement: Turn the Chair Left 90 Degrees (Figures 5-10 to 5-12)

The purpose of this transition is to make the wheelchair movement a part of your Tai Chi Chuan movement.

From the position in figure 5-9, as you rotate the torso to the right, press your left hand slightly out and up, and swing out the right arm to the right in an upward curve across the forehead, palm facing out, right hand slightly higher than the left (figure 5-10).

As the torso turns 45 degrees to the right, both hands float down to the top of the wheels and hold the hand rims to prepare for a 90-degree turn to the left (figure 5-11).

Complete the 90-degree left turn with both hands holding on to the hand rims (figure 5-12).

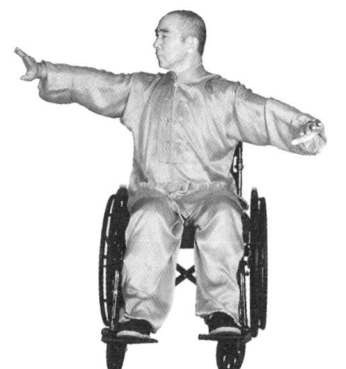 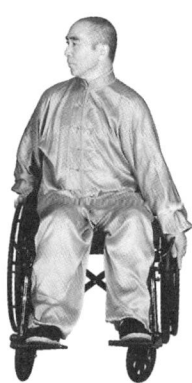 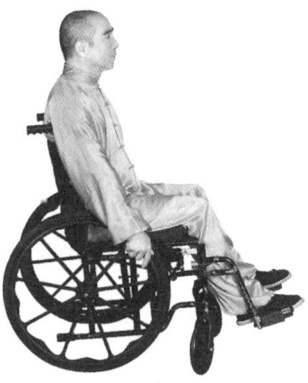

Figure 5-10   Figure 5-11   Figure 5-12

Helpful pointers: The holding position: To make the 90-degree turn, the left hand holds the left hand rim at the slight-left top, and the right hand holds the slightly back top of the right hand rim.

Become one: Make sure that the chair movement is synchronized with the body movements before and after.

The chair has your back. During the turning motion, be sure that your back firmly presses against the back of the chair. Try to avoid shifting and rocking the body.

INSIGHTS

The turning of the chair is a circular motion. The first part of the circle (figures 5-9 to 5-11) is a process of yielding by embracing an external force through a circular movement (turning the body and arms to hold the wheels). The second part of the circle (figures 5-11 to 5-12) is powerfully redirecting the circle (the turning of the chair). Thus, this movement synthesizes the motions of the body, the emotions, and the chair, transforming their relationship.

Movement 3: Grasp the Bird's Tail (Figures 5-12 to 5-20)

Grasp the Bird's Tail is a unique extended movement in Tai Chi Chuan. It consists of the four basic energies of engagement: expanding energy (掤, *Peng*), rolling back energy (捋, *Lu*), pressing or squeezing energy (挤, *Ji*), and pushing downward energy (按, *An*). The steps of this movement below also highlight the beginning and end of each of these four energies.

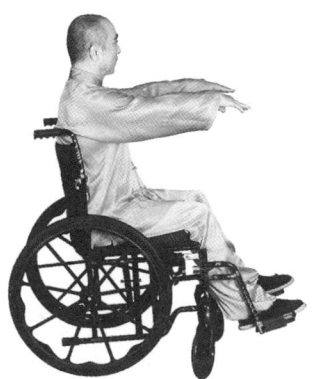

Figure 5-13

Ward Off with Both Arms (*Peng*) (Figures 5-12 to 5-13)

As you rotate the torso 45 degrees to the left, lift both arms upward and gently leftward to shoulder height and shoulder width (ward-off energy). Keep the elbows slightly bent and pointed downward and look toward the hands (figure 5-13).

Rolling Back (*Lu*) (Figures 5-13 to 5-15)

As you turn the torso slightly to the left, extend the left hand forward and turn the right palm to face upward through a small circle, placing it at the underside of the left wrist (figure 5-14). As the torso turns 45 degrees to the right, both arms roll downward and outward across the knees to the right side of the body; the gaze follows the hands (figure 5-15).

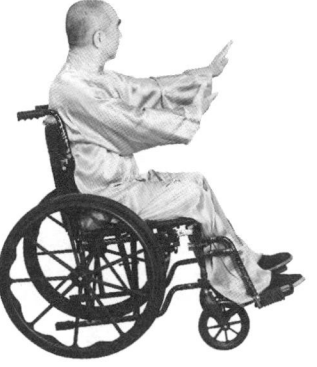

Figure 5-14

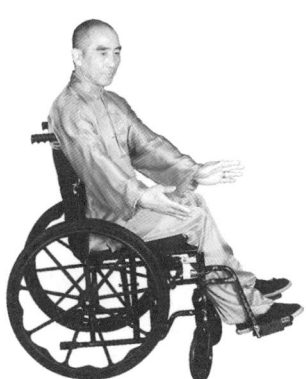

Figure 5-15

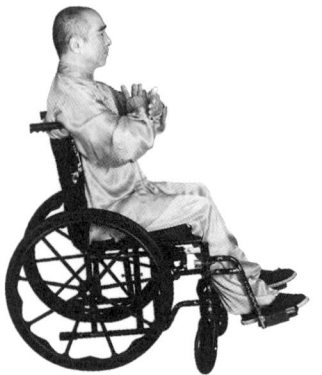

Figure 5-16

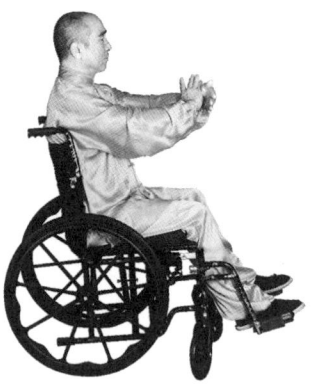

Figure 5-17

Press (*Ji*) (Figures 5-15 to 5-17)

Continue the circular motion and swing both hands outward and upward, passing the side of your right shoulder. Place the left arm crossing the chest with the palm facing the chest and the pinky edge of the right hand touching the inside of the left wrist, palm forward. Gaze forward and be ready to press the left hand outward (figure 5-16).

As the right hand presses the left inner wrist forward to form a circle with the arms at shoulder height, keep the body upright and slightly pressed backward. Both elbows point down; the eyes gaze forward (pressing energy) (figure 5-17).

Push (*An*) (Figures 5-17 to 5-20)

As you extend both hands forward, the right hand crosses over the left. Turn both palms face down and open them to shoulder width and height (figure 5-18).

Bend the elbows down and curl the hands, then draw them back to the chest, palms face down (figure 5-19).

Without stopping, push the hands down to the front of the abdomen and then push out, curving up and forward. Both palms face forward and are at shoulder height and width (pushing energy) (figure 5-20).

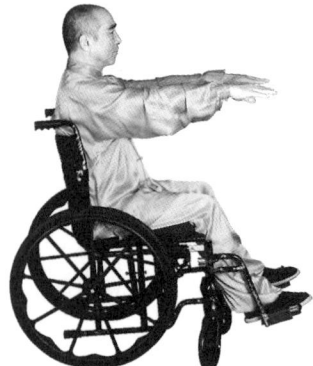

Figure 5-18

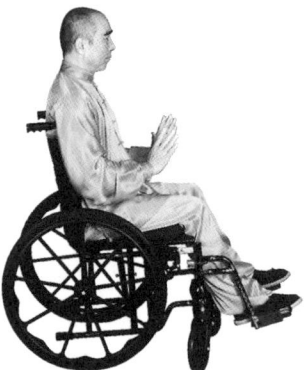

Figure 5-19

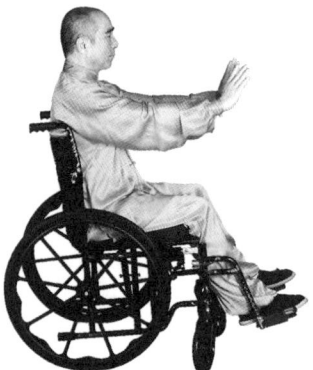

Figure 5-20

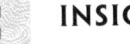

INSIGHTS

Grasping the Bird's Tail is a unique movement in Tai Chi Chuan. Within one big circular movement are four smaller circles, each of which illustrates a way of engagement.

Ward off: The first half of the circle of *Peng* energy (figures 5-9 to 5-12) includes the turning of the wheelchair. This circular movement channels an external force by bringing it close to your center. This energy can then transform into the force that turns the chair. The energy generated through this process becomes the source of power for warding off (figures 5-12 to 5-13).

Rollback: The first half of the circle of *Lu* (figures 5-13 to 5-14) is to create the momentum for the second half by following the external force and then changing its direction with a small circular turn. The second part of the circle (figures 5-14 to 5-15) redirects that force with a waterfall motion.

Press: The first half of the circle of *Ji* (figures 5-15 to 5-16) is to bring the external force close to your center (mind and body) through a circling-up movement. This yielding movement generates compressed energy in the torso, which transforms into the source of power for the final pressing-out movement (figures 5-16 to 5-17).

Push: The first half of the circle of *An* (figures 5-18 to 5-19) is to channel an incoming force close to your center by using an up-down curve. Like the energy of *pressing* above, the motion of two hands rolling back, which channels the incoming external force close to your center, also generates compressed energy in your torso. This energy transforms into power for completing the second part of the circle to push out the external force (figures 5-19 to 5-20).

The use of four energies in one circular motion demonstrates that changes and challenges are constant and unavoidable, but the ways we have to work with them can always be transformed. Different challenges tend to give birth to different solutions, and vice versa.

Helpful pointers: Ward off (*Peng*): The energy of lifting the arms in an upward and forward circle needs to come from the feeling of the body sinking. Imagine that the arms are becoming connected with the feet and you use power from the rooted feet to gently ward off a force.

Rollback (*Lu*): The rollback motion should be smooth and controlled, like water flowing downhill. The rollback movement needs to be led by the turning and shifting of the body.

Pressing (*Ji*): The energy of pressing forward should come from the motions of the body sinking and pressing back gently.

Push (*An*): The movement of bringing the hands back (figures 5-18 to 5-19), bringing them down, and pushing them out (figures 5-19 to 5-20) is a waving circle, like redirecting a moving wave. When practicing this movement, be sure to relax the upper body, including the arms, and avoid rocking the upper body forward and backward.

⦂ Transitional Movement: Roll the Chair Forward (Figures 5-20 to 5-24)

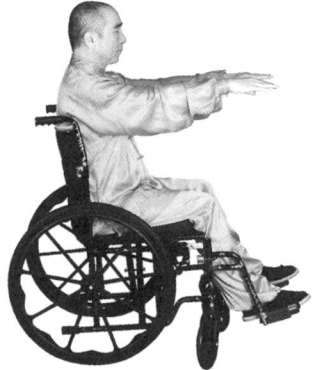

Figure 5-21

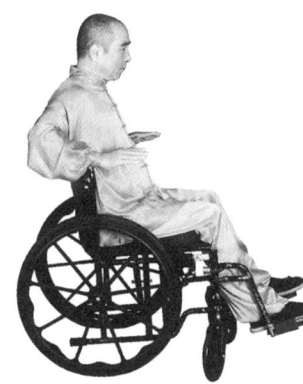

Figure 5-22

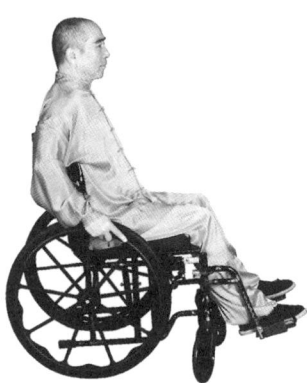

Figure 5-23

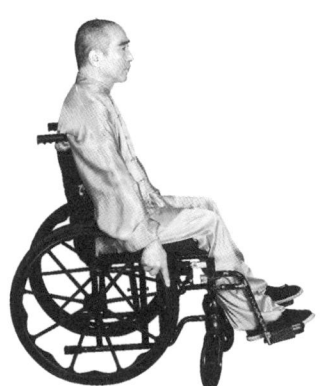

Figure 5-24

From the position in figure 5-20, place both palms face down. Bring them back toward the shoulder and then push them down to hold the top hand rims of the wheelchair (figures 5-20 to 5-23).

Push your hands to roll the chair forward about 3 to 4 feet; stop rolling with both hands holding the hand rims (figure 5-24).

Helpful pointers: Unify the motions: After pushing the wheels forward, keep both hands loosely on the hand rims and stop the forward motion by holding the hand rims.

Synchronization: Make sure that the forward motion of the wheelchair aligns with the rhythms of the moves before and after the chair's moving.

The chair has your back: While pushing the chair forward, your back presses firmly against the back; avoid shifting and rocking the body.

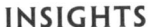

INSIGHTS

Moving the chair forward is also a circular movement. The first part of the circle (figures 5-20 to 5-23), moving your hands back in an up-down curve, yields to an incoming external force by bringing it close to the center; the second part of the circle (figures 5-23 to 5-24) redirects the force with a circular and rolling-out motion.

As prescribed by the principles of Tai Chi Chuan, the end of one movement prepares for the beginning of the next. Thus, moving the chair forward extends the previous movement and sets up the momentum for the beginning of the next.

In this context, rolling the chair forward also gives the practitioner a sense of expanded space and mobility and transforms the wheelchair from an assistive device to a tool for creating power.

Movement 4: Lift the Sky and Push the Earth (Figures 5-24 to 5-28)

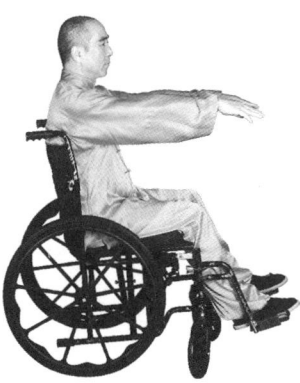

Figure 5-25

Use the momentum of the wheelchair rolling forward to float both hands straight up to shoulder height and width (figure 5-25).

As you turn the torso 45 degrees to the right, swing both arms 45 degrees to the right. While the right hand continues to circle down to the side of the right hip, palm facing up, bend the left arm and cross it in front of the chest, palm facing down, and looking straight ahead (figure 5-26).

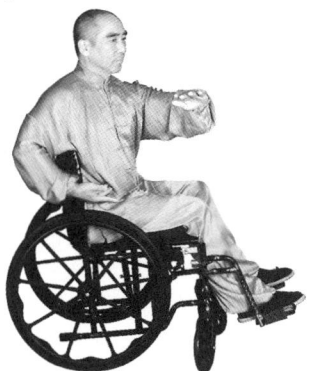

Figure 5-26

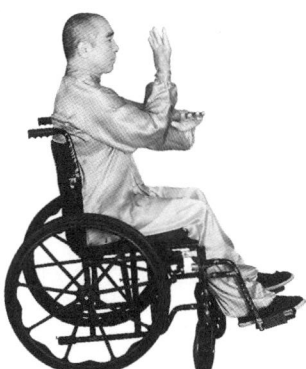

Figure 5-27

Fold the body slightly as the right palm shoots upward inside the left arm, with the left palm facing down and the right facing inward (figure 5-27).

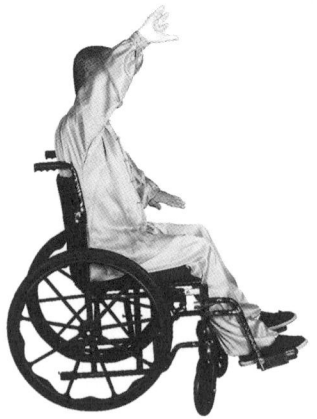

Figure 5-28

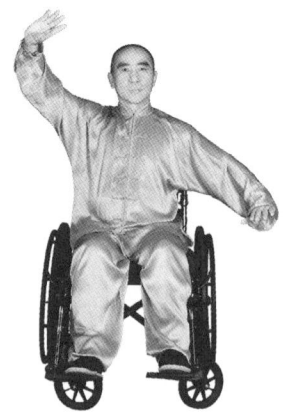

Figure 5-28a

Unfold your body as you drive the right elbow upward to the right and roll the right palm facing up; at the same time, push the left palm down and out to the left side facing downward (figures 5-28 to 5-28B).

Helpful pointers: To fold is to unfold: When moving into the position in figure 5-27, slightly fold your body while keeping the body upright. This provides the energy for the opening motion.

The chair has your back: When folding and unfolding your body, be sure that your back is firmly against the back of the chair. Not only will your body have good support, but it will also transform the back of the chair into a source of power.

Adaptation: For those who find it challenging to raise the arms above the shoulder, instead of pushing the right hand upward, you could push it forward at chest height.

To sit is to rise: When using either method, the pushing or expanding effect should be driven by the energy from the low back/chair; try to avoid tensing up the shoulder, arms, and chest.

⠿ Transitional Movement: Turn the Chair Left 180 Degrees (Figures 5-29 to 5-31)

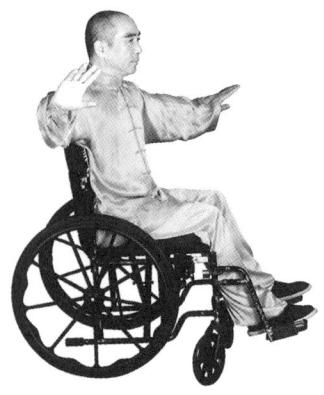

Figure 5-29

From the position in figure 5-28, as you turn the torso 45 degrees to the right, open your arms to the sides (figure 5-29).

Both hands flow down and hold the hand rims of the chair, with the right hand holding the back top of the right hand rim and the left holding the front top of the left hand rim (figure 5-30).

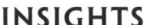

INSIGHTS

This movement originated from Chen-style Tai Chi Chuan, where this movement is called "Golden Rooster Stands on One Leg."

The first part of the circle, starting with the pushing chair motion, is to flow with the external force and bring it close to one's center through a circular yielding motion (figures 5-21 to 5-26). The second part of the circle applies the energy one generated through yielding to redirect that force (figures 5-26 to 5-28).

This movement offers a powerful lesson in flow. Imagine if one stops the movement in the position illustrated in figure 5-27. The compressed energy generated through the folding process would transform into a constraining force that makes one feel like one is being tied up, contained, restrained, or stuck. However, if you continue the movement and keep flowing, the folding position will transform into a powerful motion.

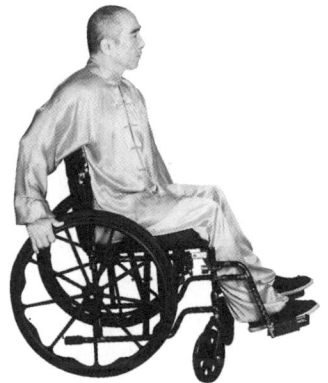

Figure 5-30

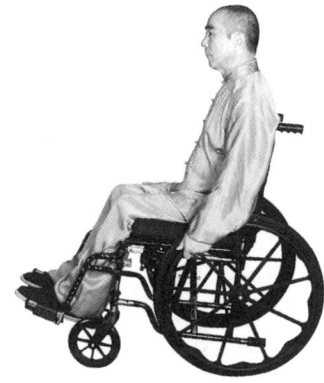

Figure 5-31

Gently make a complete 180-degree turn to the left with a flowing motion (figure 5-31).

Helpful pointers: Make the 180-degree turn: when making the turn, hold and push down the left hand rim as the right hand focuses more on the turning motion.

Synchronization: Make sure that the turning of the chair is synchronized to the movements before and after the chair turning.

The chair has your back: During the turning motion, be sure that your back presses against the back of the chair firmly to avoid body shifting and rocking.

INSIGHTS

This turning movement gives practitioners a sense of unity (of chair, practitioner, and movement) and the power to make the change through gentle, flowing, and circular motion. It also provides the momentum for the next movement.

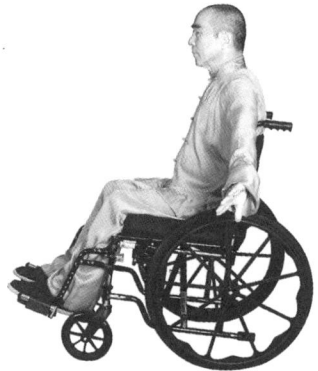

Figure 5-32

Movement 5: Flying Arrow Chases the Tiger, or Cover Hand and Thrust Fist (Figures 5-31 to 5-35)

From the position in figure 5-31, let both hands gently flow away and upward from the sides of the wheels, with palms facing back (figure 5-32).

The arms continue to swing up in an outward circular movement; as the hands approach shoulder level, turn the palms upward and bring the arms together in front of you in a "V" shape slightly above chest height, bend the elbows, and press firmly against the back of the chair (figure 5-33).

While turning the torso 45 degrees to the left, pull the left hand back and simultaneously make a loose fist facing up, and place the pinky side of your fist against the belly button. At the same time, move the right arm inward slightly to the front of the centerline, creating a gentle blocking energy, with palm facing up and at nose height (figure 5-34).

As you turn the torso 45 degrees to the right, quickly but gently pull the right palm back and make a loose fist that replaces the left fist. At the same time, roll the left fist over and punch it out over the right forearm to nose height (figure 5-35).

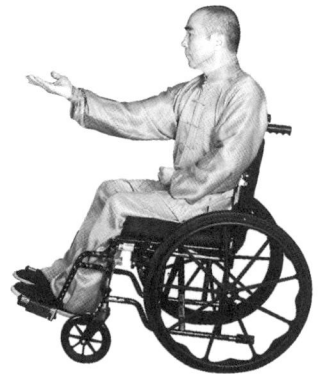
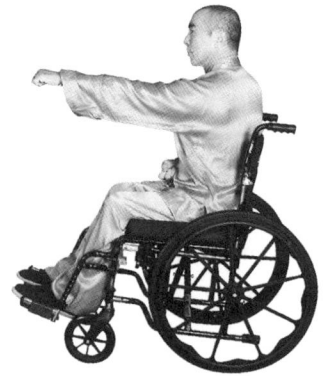

Figure 5-33

Figure 5-34 (right)
Figure 5-35 (far right)

Helpful pointers: Modification: If raising the forearms above the shoulder becomes challenging, you can form the "V" shape (figure 5-33) at chest height, keeping both elbows pointing down and at a low chest height in front of the body.

Make the chair the source of power: When throwing the left fist out, encourage the body to sink down and keep it upright, letting the energies generated by the body sink too. Pressing against the back of the chair drives the pull of the right hand back and the punch of the left fist out.

Flow like an arrow: Avoid tensing up the left arm and fist when punching; keep the fist loose and visualize your left fist as an arrow and the energy created by pulling your right hand back as the bow.

Have a focus: Let the arrow soar through an imagined target in front of you.

INSIGHTS

In Chen-style Tai Chi Chuan, this movement is called "Cover Hand and Thrust Fist." In Chen style, the expression of energies or forces varies according to the context, unlike in other styles of Tai Chi Chuan. In Yang style, for example, the expression of redirecting energy is always slow and gentle, like the slow motion of a wave. In Chen style, redirecting energy can be expressed in quite an explosive way, like a lightning bolt in a thunderstorm. In this movement (figures 5-32 to 5-34), the motion for the first part of the circle is slow and fluid; the motion for the second part of the circle, however, is quick and explosive. Many practitioners enjoy this movement because it provides them with an experiential understanding of the power of yielding. Plus it's exciting!

In external martial arts, one usually punches *at* something. However, in Tai Chi Chuan, one punches *through* something. To punch through something requires calm, focused, and expanded mental space, as when shooting an arrow from a bow. That is why this movement is called "Flying Arrow Chases the Tiger."

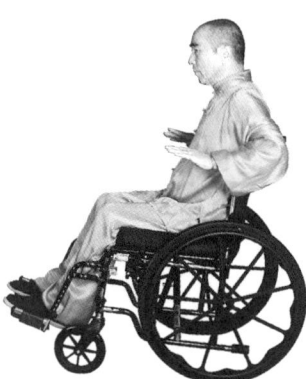

Figure 5-36

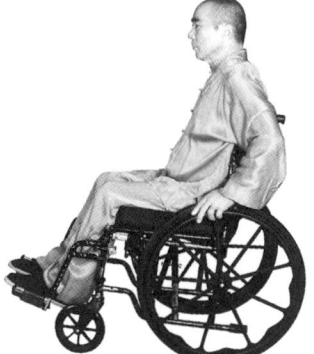

Figure 5-37

⁞ Transitional Movement: Hold and Move the Wheels Forward (Figures 5-35 to 5-40)

From the position in figure 5-35, as your torso turns to face front, slowly slide the right fist along the underside of the left forearm to cross at the wrists, with the right fist facing up and the left facing down (figure 5-36).

Slowly open the fists and raise the arms so both hands are at shoulder height, palms facing up (figure 5-37).

While turning both palms face down, bring the arms back in a curve to the position above the wheels (figure 5-38).

Hold the hand rims of the chair from the top and move the chair forward 3 to 4 feet in slow motion (figures 5-39 to 5-40).

Helpful pointers: Make the chair's motion a part of the movement: after pushing the wheels forward, keep both hands loosely on the hand rims and stop the forward motion by holding the hand rims.

Connecting the rhythms: Make sure that the motion of the wheelchair moving forward synchronizes with the rhythms of the moves before and after.

Chair and body become one: While pushing the chair forward, your back presses against the back of the chair firmly to avoid shifting and rocking the body.

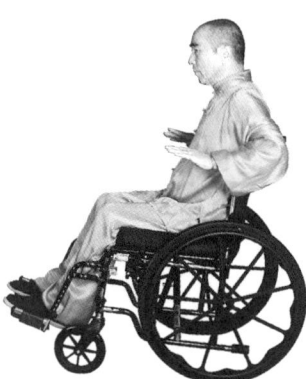

Figure 5-38

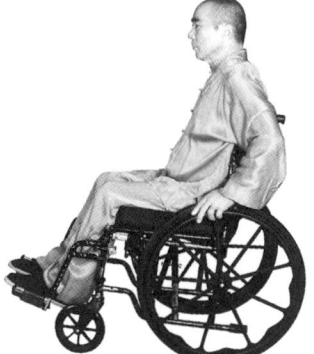

Figure 5-39

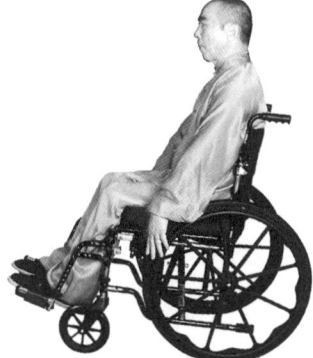

Figure 5-40

INSIGHTS

Moving the chair forward is also a circular movement. The first part of the circle (figures 5-35 to 5-39) is to yield to an incoming force and bring it closer to the center; the second part of the circle (figures 5-39 to 5-40) is to redirect the force by using a circular and rolling-out motion. In addition, the momentum or energy generated by moving the chair forward provides power for the next movement. In Tai Chi Chuan, the end of one circle is the beginning of the next. The movement of rolling the chair forward gives the practitioner a sense of expansion and mobility. It also transforms the wheelchair from an assistive device into a tool for creating power.

Movement 6: Needle at the Bottom of the Ocean (Figures 5-40 to 5-48)

From the position in figure 5-40, slowly float your hands away from the wheels to shoulder height and width, with palms facing down (figure 5-41).

Slowly bend the elbows and turn the palms to face forward as you curve the arms back to the front of the chest (figure 5-42).

Drop the elbows down slightly and push both palms forward in a slight curving-up motion, with palms facing forward and elbows slightly bent (figure 5-43).

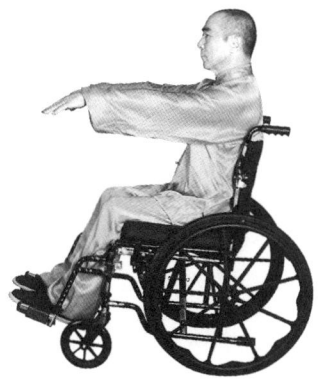

Figure 5-41

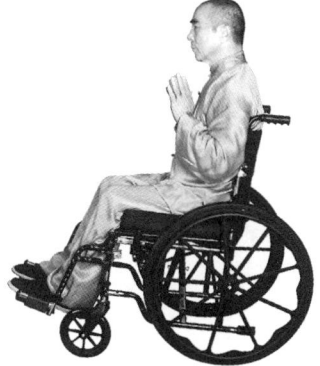

Figure 5-42

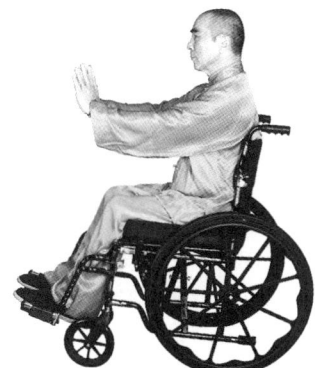

Figure 5-43

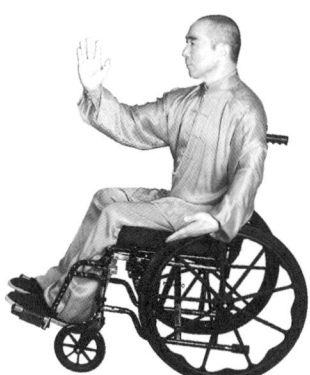

Figure 5-44

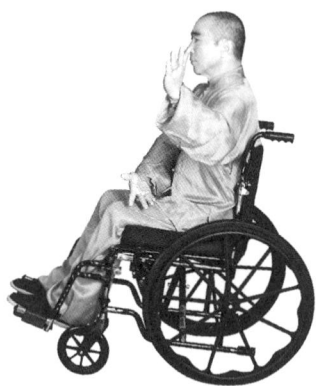

Figure 5-45

While turning the torso 45 degrees to the left, drop the left arm down and pull the left palm to the side of the hip with the palm facing up. Simultaneously, bend your right elbow a little more and let the right palm move across the center line to the left, palm facing left and at shoulder height (figure 5-44).

As you swing the left hand in the outward and upward curve to the front of your left shoulder with the palm facing right, the right hand continues the blocking motion downward to the position above the left knee, the palm facing up (figure 5-45).

As the torso turns 45 degrees to the right, guide the right hand across the knees and swing it out and upward to the right side of the body, palm facing up, while the left hand moves across the face to the right (figure 5-46).

As the right hand continues to float up at the side of the body, passing the shoulder and arriving at the side of the head, thumb pointing up and palm facing the right temple, the left hand circles down to the right side of the hip with fingers pointing slightly down (figure 5-47).

While turning the torso 45 degrees to the left, move the left hand across the front of the knees to the left side of the wheel with the palm facing down (blocking-away energy), and strike the right hand down to the left, with the thumb pointing up and fingers pointing 45 degrees downward (figure 5-48).

Helpful pointers: The revolving door effect: Turn the body like a revolving door and keep the body upright.

Yin and yang: As the body turns to the left, let the left hand lead (yin) the right hand (yang), and vice versa.

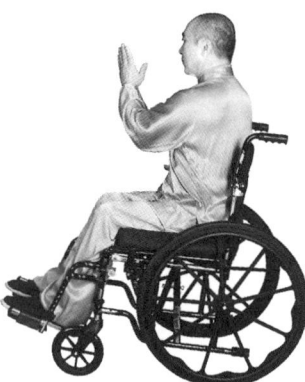

Figure 5-46

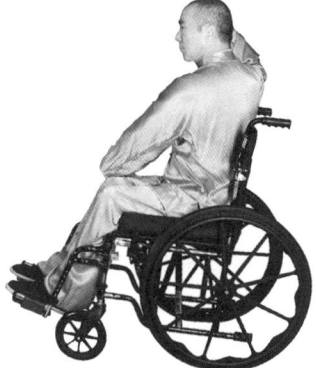

Figure 5-47

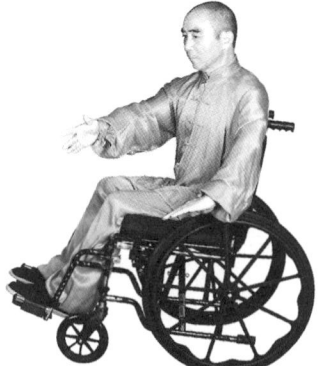

Figure 5-48

INSIGHTS

The first two turning movements are to block or deflect an incoming force through the revolving-door energy. They oppose the "wax-on" and "wax-off" movement. "Wax on, wax off," a phrase that became popular from the 1984 movie *The Karate Kid*, refers to a martial arts deflecting movement that makes a clockwise vertical circle with the right hand and a counterclockwise vertical circle with the left. This movement is similar to the Tai Chi movement "cloud hands." The second part of the circle (figures 5-47 to 5-48) is the striking-down motion driven by the energy generated through the two blocking movements.

Body and chair become one: While turning the body slowly, press the back against the chair and keep the body upright.

The chair has your back: When striking down the right palm to the left, keep the back against the back of the chair.

Mental focus: When striking the right hand down to a 45-degree low left angle, visualize your palm, like a spear, striking down to strike a fish at the bottom of the ocean.

Transitional Movement: Hold and Turn the Wheels to the Left 90 Degrees (Figures 5-49 to 5-51)

From the position in figure 5-48, as you rotate the torso to the right, push your left hand slightly out and up and swing the right arm out to the right in an up-and-down curve across the forehead, palm facing out, right hand slightly higher than the left (figure 5-49).

As the torso turns 45 degrees to the right, both hands float down to the top of the wheels and hold the hand rims to prepare for a 90-degree turn to the left (figure 5-50).

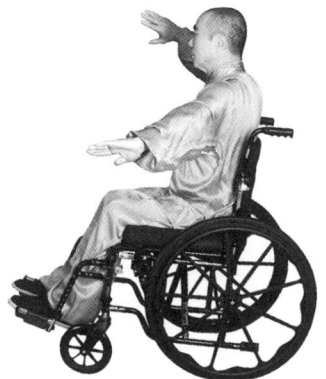

Figure 5-49

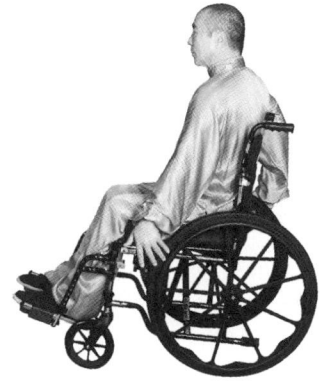

Figure 5-50

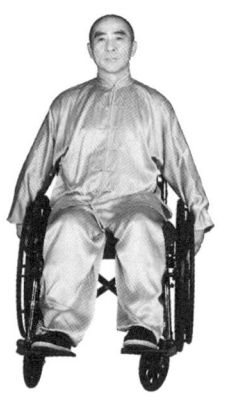

Figure 5-51

Stop the turning motion after the 90-degree left turn is complete, with both hands holding the hand rims (figure 5-51).

Helpful pointers: The holding position: to make the 90-degree turn, the left hand holds the left top rim slightly to the front and the right hand holds the right top rim slightly to the back.

Become one: Make sure that the chair's movement is smooth and synchronized with the moves before and after the turning.

The chair has your back: While turning, be sure that your back firmly presses against the chair to avoid shifting and rocking.

INSIGHTS

The turning of the chair is circular. The first part of the circle (figures 5-48 to 5-50) is a process of yielding by embracing an external force through turning the body and arms; the second part of the circle (figures 5-50 to 5-51) is to redirect an external force through turning the chair. The turning of the chair also generates momentum for the next movement. Thus, this movement synergizes the motions of the practitioner's body, mind, and chair and transforms the function of the wheelchair.

Movement 7: Bend the Bow to Shoot the Tiger (Figures 5-51 to 5-54)

While rotating the torso 45 degrees to the left, lift both arms upward and leftward to shoulder height and width (ward-off energy). Keep the elbows slightly bent and look toward your hands (figure 5-52).

While turning the torso 45 degrees to the right, roll the arms downward to the right with palms facing down. When both hands circle up to the right side of the head, make fists and bend both elbows. Place the left fist in front of the right elbow, with the heart of the right fist facing up slightly and the heart of the left fist facing right (figure 5-53).

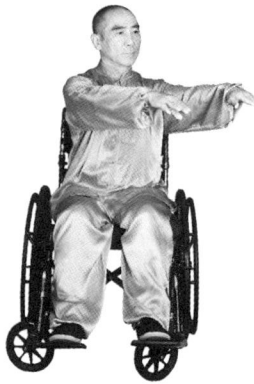

Figure 5-52

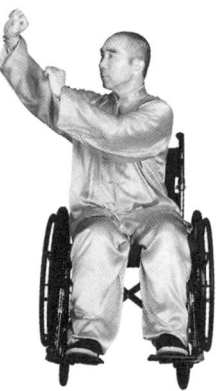

Figure 5-53

Slightly turn the body to the left while striking both fists 45 degrees out to the left. The right fist is slightly above the right forehead and the left fist is away from the body at nose height with the elbow bent (figure 5-54).

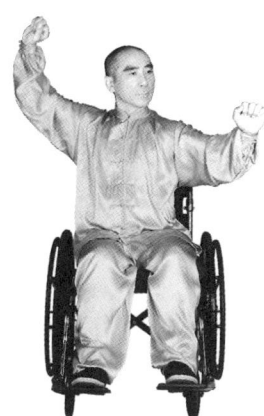

Figure 5-54

Helpful pointers: Become one: the upward warding-off movement needs to link with the rhythm of the chair turning.

Flow like water: Rolling down after the warding-off movement is flowing and circular, like a waterfall.

Sit like a mountain: When turning the body to strike, make sure that the energies come from the body's sinking and pressing against the back of the chair while turning.

The chair has your back: When punching, be sure that your back is pressing against the chair.

Modification: If you feel discomfort when raising the right arm high, you can lower the right hand to any level you find comfortable.

INSIGHTS

Practicing this movement always conjures the image of hunters on horseback using bows and arrows. The swing of both arms to the left after turning the chair is the energy of warding off, then it changes to rollback energy as you roll the hands down and across the knees to the right. Finally, the rollback motion cultivates the energy of "bend the bow to shoot the tiger."

Most important, sinking into the chair and making the turn gives more power to the striking movement. Therefore, the chair transforms into a dynamic power source for the movement.

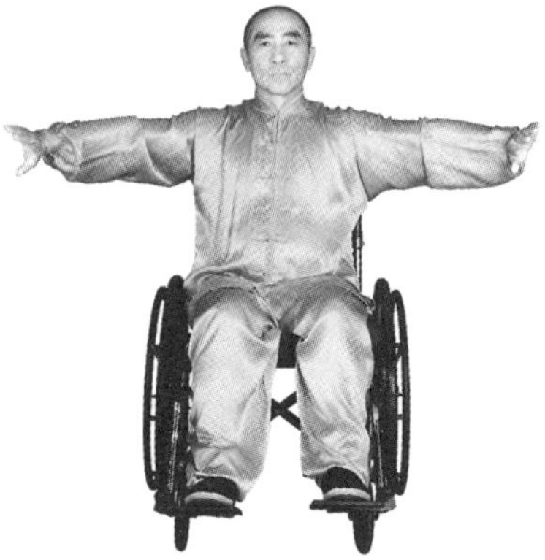

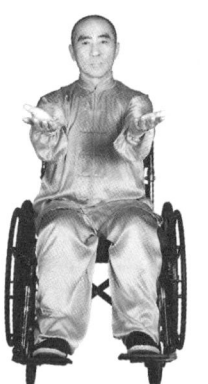

Figure 5-55

⦂ Closing Form (Figures 5-54 to 5-63)

From the position in figure 5-54, rotate the body facing front while extending arms out to the side at shoulder level, palms facing out (figure 5-55).

As palms turn to face up, bring the arms to the front of the chest in a circular motion; both hands are shoulder width and slightly below shoulder height (figure 5-56).

Gently pull the arms back to the sides of the hips, palms facing up (figure 5-57).

Swing the arms out and up to shoulder height and turn palms to face

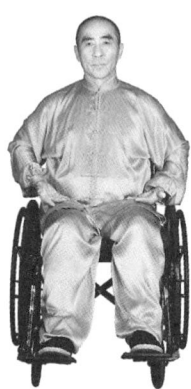

Figure 5-56

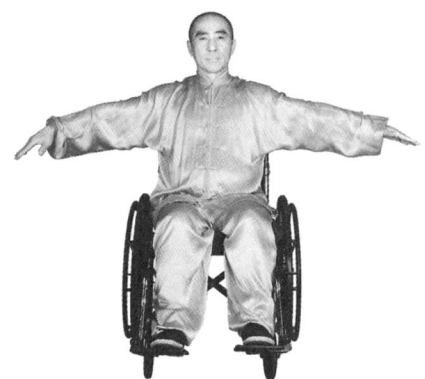

Figure 5-57

Figure 5-58

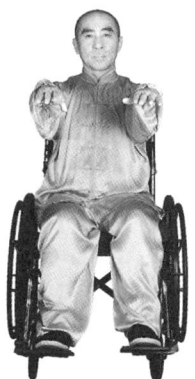

Figure 5-59

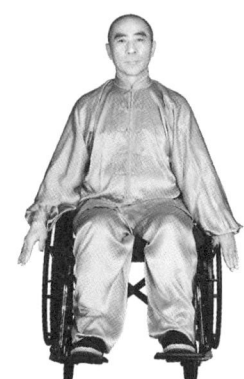

Figure 5-60

down (figure 5-58).

Bring both hands to the front; keep the arms at shoulder width and height, palms face down (figure 5-59).

Gently bring both hands down to the outside of the wheels (figure 5-60).

Slowly lift the arms up from the sides, palms up; turn the palms facing down when both hands reach the front top of the forehead, and then gently push the hands down to the outside of the wheels (figures 5-61 to 5-63).

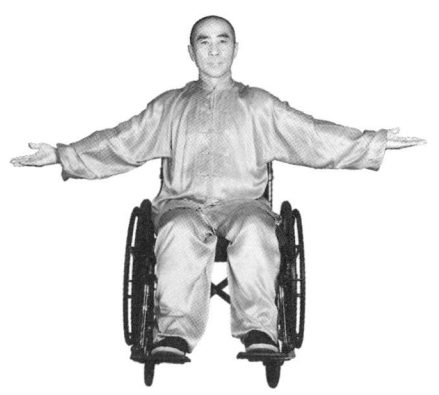

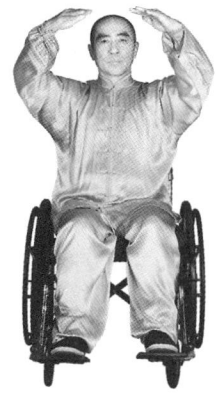

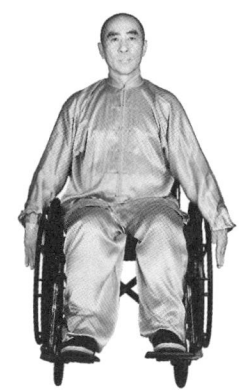

| Figure 5-61 | Figure 5-62 | Figure 5-63 |

Helpful pointers: Body moves arms: When extending arms out at shoulder height, be sure that the arm movement synchronizes with the motion of rotating the body (figures 5-54 to 5-55).

Synchronization: When bringing both hands from the sides of the shoulder to the front, synchronize the turning of the arms and the palms to face up (figures 5-55 to 5-56).

Relax the shoulders: Avoid tensing up the shoulders when pulling the arms back and swing them out to the front, alongside the hips (figures 5-56 to 5-58).

Modification: For those who find raising the arms above the shoulders challenging (figure 5-62), you can adjust the arms up to a comfortable height—to the height of the chest, for example.

A big circle: The entire closing movement is a big circle with a few turns. Making the motion flow like a gentle stream creates a calming sense of focus and closure.

Take a moment: After bringing the arms down to the sides, sit for a few seconds before moving on to your next activity.

THE COMMENCING AND CLOSING FORMS

All Tai Chi Chuan sequences have a ritualistic opening and closing form. The opening form is a preparatory physical stance for a calm mind, centered body, and mindful breathing. It is the foundation for the flow of energy and movements that follow—the commencing movements—and is essential to your practice. The transition from the preparatory posture to the commencing movement is a significant transition from the state of readiness (Wu Chi) to the statement of engagement (Tai Chi). The commencing movement is the beginning of cultivating energy/Qi/power through purposeful and flowing movements. The closing form helps practitioners to ground themselves and return to a calm, centered, and balanced state after the dynamic movements.

Such ritual forms or structures are seen in all martial arts and in public events such as festivals, celebrations, and artistic performances. They function as a rite of passage. According to cultural anthropologists, rites of passage are universal cultural practices throughout human history and across all ethnic groups. They are effective ways for humans to make sense of crises and mentally prepare themselves for challenges. Most rites of passage—such as the celebration of a birth, the transition from puberty to adulthood, marriage, military enlistment, or graduation—have three distinct stages: separation, transition, and incorporation.

We can view the opening form (separation) of a Tai Chi Chuan practice as an important way to signify one's entrance (transition) into a new realm that represents positive changes. The closing form signifies the end of this process and the readiness to re-engage in social life (incorporation).

6

Stand Like a Tree and Flow Like a River
Standing Tai Chi Chuan

I N MARTIAL ARTS, all body stances and forms can be points of engagement once you let your body become the mind and the mind become the body. This enlightened realization comes from observing nature. In nature, no one thing or object is more powerful than the rest, and everything serves a function in its own ecological niche. Such balanced relationships create a powerful and sustainable natural environment. Deeply rooted trees do not give us a sense of immobility or limitation. Quite the opposite, deeply rooted trees manifest uprising, flowing energies that give us a sense of inspiration, power, centeredness, beauty, and flexibility.

Centered, flowing engagement is the way of Tai Chi Chuan movements, and it is the way of a tree and a metaphor for everything in nature. The movement title "Stand Like a Tree and Move Like a River" (1) emphasizes the relationship between the way of nature and the way of the human body, (2) illustrates that opposites create unity and that rooting creates energy that rises up, and (3) promotes a mind-centered engagement that empowers both mind and body.

Who benefits from this modality? The seven postures of standing Tai Chi Chuan are suitable for everyone, including those with ambulatory conditions. The practice is accessible and can effectively engage the mind and body with practically no environmental constraints or space limitations. One can practice at home or in an office or hotel room while standing in front of a window and looking out at a tree, pond, or garden.

This modality can also be an ideal fitness or rehabilitation tool for folks with limited ambulatory mobility. I learned from healthcare providers at VA medical centers across the country that the standing modality is one of their most popular forms of Tai Chi Chuan practices. Many ambulatory veterans were reluctant to participate in any physical fitness or sports program because of injuries or joint conditions, but have found that standing Tai Chi Chuan is an easier and accessible practice that improves their physical and mental health.

The central idea of this modality is not just about practicing Tai Chi Chuan in the standing position but about making the standing posture part of the flowing energy of Tai Chi Chuan. One of the key elements for achieving a centered, flowing engagement is to make the centered lower body the driving force for the upward-flowing movements. To achieve this, the standing modality has four unique requirements:

> In one of the Wheelchair Tai Chi virtual classes, a Vietnam veteran from Wisconsin started the practice in a wheelchair. A few years later, he practices while standing in front of a walker.

1. *Awareness of the body's center:* Always be aware of the body's center and keep it upright throughout the practice. Aristotle said, "Knowing yourself is the beginning of all wisdom." In the context of Tai Chi Chuan practice, yourself is the body center. Therefore, knowing is letting the mind know or become a part of the center of your body.

2. *Engaging 45 degrees of rotation:* The phrase "rotating and turning the body 45 degrees" left or right is used to guide the body as it turns. Though the degree of the rotation depends on the condition of the body, it emphasizes the importance of initiating each movement through the torso or the lower back.

3. *Shifting the body center:* Another important focus in this modality is shifting the body center in each move. Shifting the body center from left to right, or vice versa, is integrated into the rotating movements. These two movements provide the driving upward-moving energy.

4. *Activating the "bow stance":* The word "shifting" above can be misinterpreted since one rarely completely shifts the center from one side to the other. There is another phrase that better presents the dynamics of this shifting movement: the bow stance. The bow stance describes what a body posture should look and feel like. Shifting the center from one side to the other is the process of forming a bow stance. For example, a right bow stance is when the practitioner has 70 percent of the weight on the right leg with the body-center line two-thirds to the right foot. While the left knee is slightly bent,

the right knee is bent a bit more, but the lower leg is vertical and the kneecap is in line with the right foot. The bow stance is often referred to as the launching stance. The energy for "launching" (the upper body) comes from the lower body's sinking effect. Moving onto the right leg, for example, creates the effect of a compressed spring.

Disclaimer: Engaging in any physical exercise can lead to injury or discomfort. These practices are not intended as medical advice or treatment or to replace medical supervision and treatment. Please consult with your primary healthcare provider before starting the practice.

⦂ Preparatory Posture (Figure 6-1)

While standing, bend your knees slightly and let the body sink downward, keeping the head, neck, and body upright and holding the head straight up as if suspended from above by a thread. Release all tension from the shoulders and arms, letting the arms hang gently at your sides. Mentally connect all relaxed body parts to your body center (spine and legs), making them a calm, engaged body system. Eyes look straight ahead, their gaze like two swords that look through everything before you.

Helpful pointers: Stand like a tree: Slightly bend your knees and sink the lower part of your body downward like a rooted tree.

Root to rise: As the lower body roots into the ground like a sturdy tree trunk, lift the upper body like flourishing tree branches that give off radiant energy.

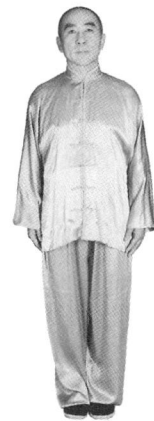

Figure 6-1

⦂ Commencement (Figures 6-2 to 6-5)

Slowly shift the body center toward the right leg and step to the left, keeping the feet close to parallel and shoulder-width apart, opening both toes slightly outward (figure 6-2).

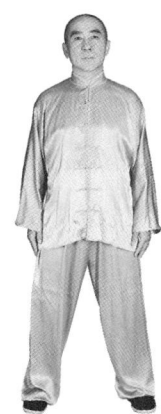

Figure 6-2

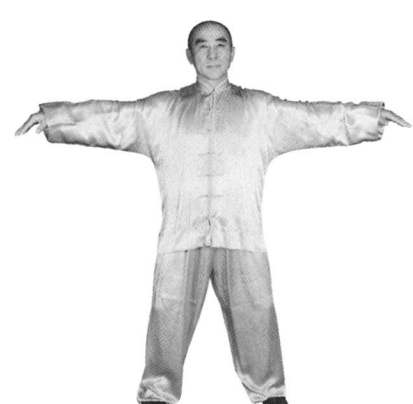

Figure 6-3

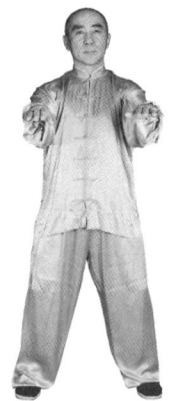

Figure 6-4

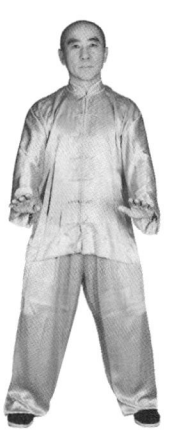

Figure 6-5

Slowly raise both arms to shoulder height, palms facing down, relaxing the wrists (figure 6-3).

Without stopping, bring the arms to the front, shoulder-width apart and shoulder height with the elbows down. Palms are relaxed and facing down (figure 6-4).

While bending your legs slowly into a comfortable position, bend and drop the elbows and draw the arms slightly inward. Push your forearms down to the front of the abdomen. Keep both hands shoulder-width apart (figure 6-5).

Helpful pointers: Opening stance: The distance between the feet (figure 6-2) can vary from one individual to the other. Once you have begun, try to stand as a rooted tree and do not move your feet during the practice.

Keeping the knees slightly bent is the key to creating a centered flow in Tai Chi Chuan practice. However, avoid bending the knees too much and moving the kneecaps freely. Two practical rules of thumb to prevent knee discomfort: always keep the kneecaps behind the toes and facing forward throughout the practice.

To stand is to rise: Imagine that the force lifting your arms comes from the lower back as your body sinks downward.

Push without pushing: When pushing your arms downward, focus on the center of the palms; imagine that you are slowly pushing a beach ball into the water.

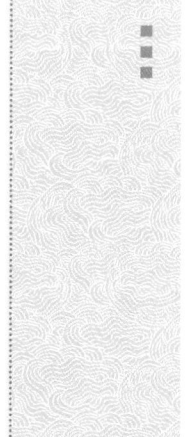

INSIGHTS

The opening movements are circular, consisting of two parts. The first part of the circle (figures 6-2 to 6-4) denotes the energy of yielding to or compiling the massive incoming forces (stressors) and bringing them close to your center; the second part of the circle (figures 6-4 to 6-5) denotes the energy of redirecting the unified force downward through a flowing movement. As you push both arms down, feel the energy of your body rising up: root to rise.

Many people like to visualize the sun rising when raising their arms and the sun setting when pushing their arms down.

⁝ Movement 1: Parting the Wild Horse's Mane
(Figures 6-6 to 6-7)

From the position in figure 6-5, shift the body center toward the left leg and slowly rotate the torso and the body 45 degrees to the left to make a left bow stance. Open both arms slightly before circling the left arm to chest height and sweeping the right hand, palm facing left, across the front of your body to the left to form the "holding a ball" position under the left arm (figure 6-6).

Rotate the torso 45 degrees to the right and shift your body center toward the right leg to make a right bow stance. Slowly push the left palm down toward the side and position the arm at the left side of the hip. At the same time, raise the right hand to chest height before swinging it out 45 degrees to the right, palm facing up. Hold the right hand just slightly below eye level (figure 6-7).

Helpful pointers: Hold a ball: When forming the "hold a ball" position (figure 6-6), keep the left palm at shoulder height and drop the elbow down; look toward the left.

Throw a frisbee: The movement of rotating the torso, shifting the center from the left leg to the right, and swinging the right hand to the right is like the movement of throwing a frisbee. Let the torso do the work and the arm follows.

Staying centered: When you are in the motion illustrated in figures 6-6 and 6-7, be sure that your body is upright and avoid leaning the body center forward or sideways.

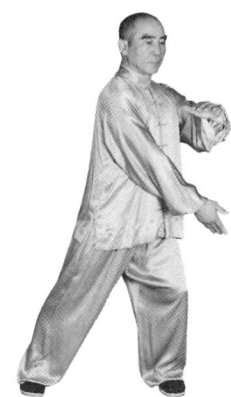

Figure 6-6

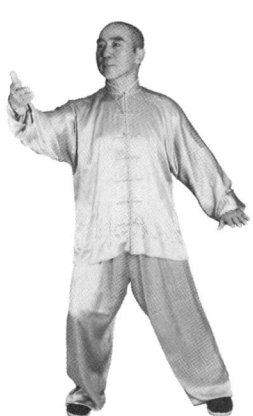

Figure 6-7

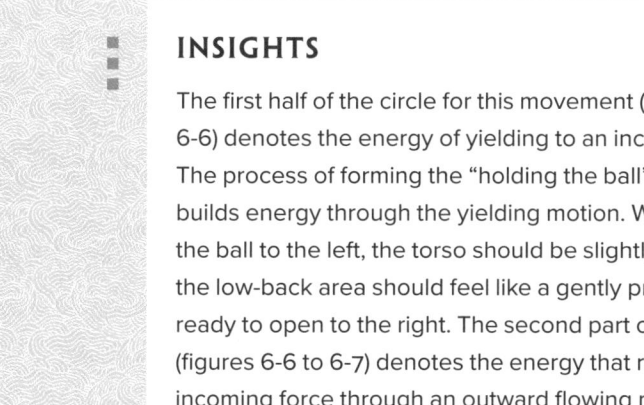

⁝ INSIGHTS

The first half of the circle for this movement (figures 6-5 to 6-6) denotes the energy of yielding to an incoming force. The process of forming the "holding the ball" position builds energy through the yielding motion. When holding the ball to the left, the torso should be slightly folded and the low-back area should feel like a gently pressed spring ready to open to the right. The second part of the circle (figures 6-6 to 6-7) denotes the energy that redirects the incoming force through an outward flowing movement.

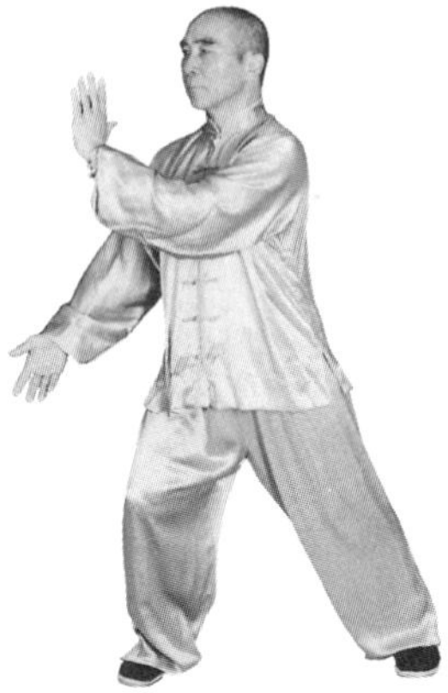

Figure 6-8

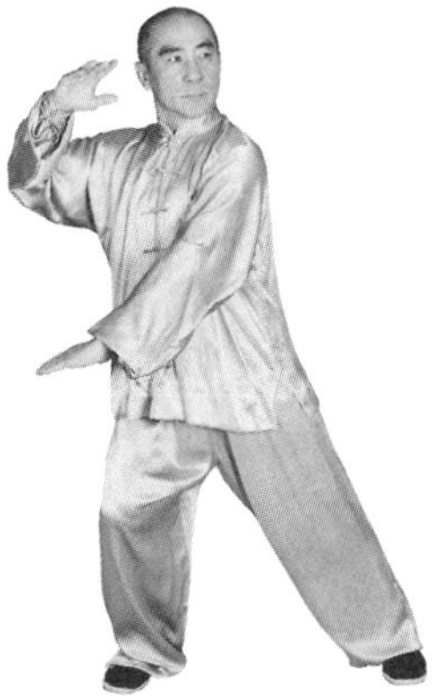

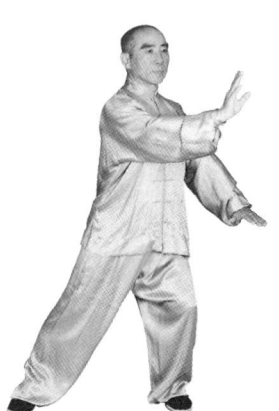

Figure 6-9

: Movement 2: Brush Knee and Push Hand
(Figures 6-7 to 6-10)

From figure 6-7, as you rotate the torso slightly to the right, glide your right hand down and to the side, with the palm facing up; at the same time, the left arm floats up to the left side of the left forehead (figure 6-8).

While keeping the body center on the right leg, the right hand, with the palm facing up, swings out and upward in a circle to the side of the right ear, changing the palm to face forward and dropping the elbow. The left arm moves to cross in front of the face, passing the right shoulder to the front of the right side of the hip (figure 6-9).

As you rotate the torso 45 degrees and shift the center to the left to make a left bow stance, sweep the left hand downward and outward across the body to the side of the left hip, with the palm facing down. Push the right hand 45 degrees to the left, with the palm facing forward and at nose height (figure 6-10).

Helpful pointers: When pushing out the right palm forward (45 degrees to the left), be sure that the energy of pushing comes from sinking the body downward.

Stay centered: When pushing (figures 6-9 and 6-10), be sure that your body is upright and avoid leaning the body center forward or sideways. Press the body slightly backward against an invisible wall behind you for added stability.

INSIGHTS

The first half of the circle for this movement (figures 6-7 to 6-9) denotes the energy of yielding to an incoming force; the second part of the circle (figures 6-9 to 6-10) denotes the energy of redirecting the incoming force through an outwardly flowing movement of the body and arms.

Figure 6-10

⁞ Movement 3: Grasp the Bird's Tail (Figures 6-10 to 6-20)

Grasp the Bird's Tail is a unique extended movement in Tai Chi Chuan. It consists of the four basic energies of engagement: expanding energy (*Peng*), rollback energy (*Lu*), pressing or squeezing energy (*Ji*), and pushing downward energy (*An*). The instructions for this movement highlight the beginning and end of each of these four energies.

Ward Off with Both Arms (*Peng*) (Figures 6-10 to 6-13)

From the position in figure 6-10, as you rotate the torso and shift the center to the right to make a right bow stance, push your left hand slightly out and swing the right arm out to the right in an up-and-down curve across the forehead. The palm faces out and the right hand is slightly higher than the left. The eyes follow the movement of the right hand, then look left (figure 6-11).

Both hands continue floating down to the sides of the hips to prepare for warding off (*Peng*) (figure 6-12).

As you rotate your torso 45 degrees to the left, shift the center toward the left leg to make a left bow stance, gently lifting both arms upward and to the left to shoulder height and at shoulder width (ward-off energy). Keep the elbows slightly bent and pointed downward. Look toward the hands (figure 6-13).

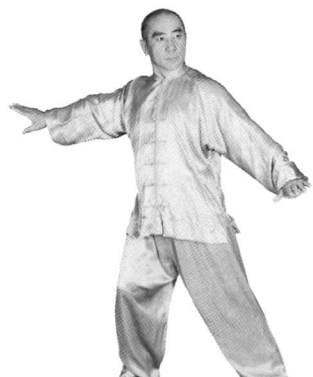 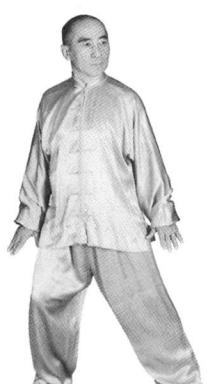 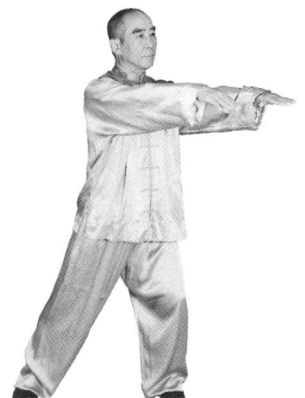

Figure 6-11   Figure 6-12   Figure 6-13

Rolling Back (*Lu*) (Figures 6-13 to 6-15)

As you turn the torso slightly to the left, extend the left hand forward and turn the right palm to face up, placing it at the underside of the left wrist (figure 6-14). As the torso turns 45 degrees to the right, shift more weight to the right leg, making a right bow stance. Both arms roll downward and outward across the abdomen to the right side of your body; eyes follow the hands (figure 6-15).

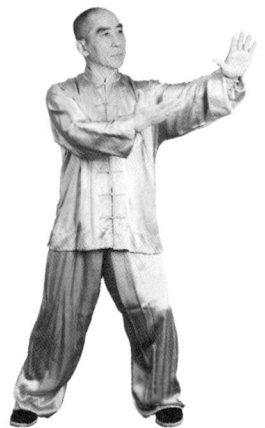
Figure 6-14

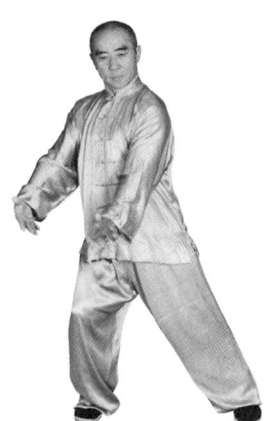
Figure 6-15

Press (*Ji*) (Figures 6-15 to 6-17)

Continue the circular motion and swing both hands out and upward, passing your right shoulder, and place the left arm across the chest with the palm facing inward and the edge of the right hand (pinky side) touching the inside of the left wrist, palm forward. Look forward and prepare to push the left hand out (figure 6-16).

As the right hand presses the left inner wrist forward so the arms form a circle at shoulder height, keep the body upright and slightly press backward; both elbows point down; look forward (pressing energy) (figure 6-17).

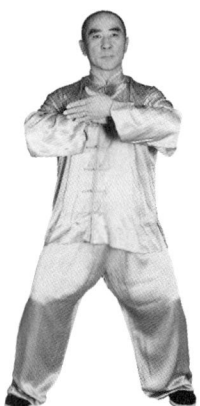
Figure 6-16

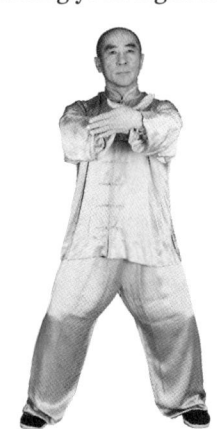
Figure 6-17

Push (An) (Figures 6-17 to 6-20)

As you extend both hands forward, the right hand crosses over the left. Turn both palms face down and open them to shoulder width and height (figure 6-18).

Bend the elbows down and draw the hands back in an up-and-down curve to the chest (figure 6-19).

Without stopping, push the hands down to the front of the abdomen and then push out with an up-and-forward curve, with both palms facing forward and at shoulder height and width (pushing energy) (figure 6-20).

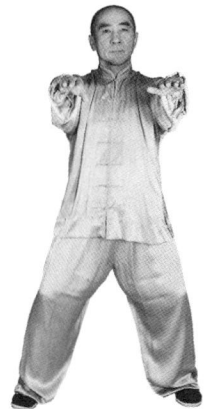
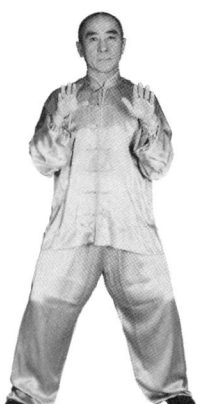
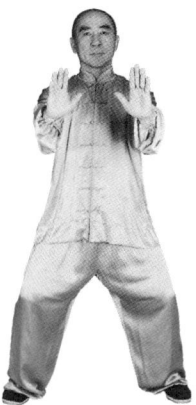

| Figure 6-18 | Figure 6-19 | Figure 6-20 |

Helpful pointers: Ward off (*Peng*): The energy of lifting the arms in an upward and forward circle needs to come from visualizing the body sinking. Imagine the arms are connected to the feet, and you use power and stability from the rooted feet to gently ward off an incoming force.

Rollback (*Lu*): The rollback motion should be smooth and controlled, like a waterfall. The rollback movement needs to be led by the turning and shifting of your body.

Pressing (*Ji*): The energy of pressing forward should come from the actions of the body sinking and pressing back gently.

Push (*An*): The movement of bringing the hands back (figures 6-18 to 6-19), pushing them down to the abdomen level, and then pushing them out (figures 6-19 to 6-20) is circular, like redirecting a wave. When practicing this movement, relax the upper body, including the arms, and avoid rocking the upper body forward and backward.

INSIGHTS

Grasping the Bird's Tail is a unique movement in Tai Chi Chuan. Within one big circular movement there are four smaller circles, each illustrating a way of engagement.

Ward off: The first half of the circle of *Peng* energy (figures 6-10 to 6-12) unifies or channels an external force by bringing it close to your center through a circular movement. In doing so, it transforms the external force into a part of the energy, which begins the second part of the circle, the ward-off movement (figures 6-12 to 6-13).

Rollback: The first half of the circle for the movement of *Lu* (figures 6-13 to 6-14) creates the momentum for the second part of the circle by following the external force and then changing its orientation by making a small circular turn; the second part of the circle (figures 6-14 to 6-15) redirects that force through a waterfall motion using the momentum generated by the first part of the circular movement.

Press: The first half of the circle for the movement of *Ji* (figures 6-15 to 6-16) brings the external force close to your center (mind and body) through a circling-up movement. This yielding movement generates compressed energy between the hands and the center of the body (figure 6-16). If the movement stops there, the compressed energy will create a negative consequence. However, if the movement continues, the compressed energy becomes a source of power for the second part of the circle, pressing that external force away (figures 6-16 to 6-17).

Push: The first half of the circle for the movement of *An* (figures 6-18 to 6-19) channels an incoming force close to your center with an up-down curve. Similar to the energy of pressing (above), the rollback motion of the hands, which channels the incoming external force close to your center, also generates compressed energy in your torso. This energy becomes the source of power, allowing the completion of the second part of the circle, which redirects the external force outward (figures 6-19 to 6-20).

Using these four types of energies in one circular motion implies that changes and challenges, and ways of working with them, are mutually inclusive or transformable energies. It also demonstrates how different changes or challenges tend to give birth to different solutions, and vice versa.

Movement 4: Hold the Sky and Push the Earth (Figures 6-20 to 6-24)

From the position in figure 6-20, turn both palms face down. As you shift the center toward the left leg and turn the torso 45 degrees to the left, bend your elbows slightly and let both arms move as you turn the torso, extending the hands slightly forward 45 degrees to the left (figure 6-21).

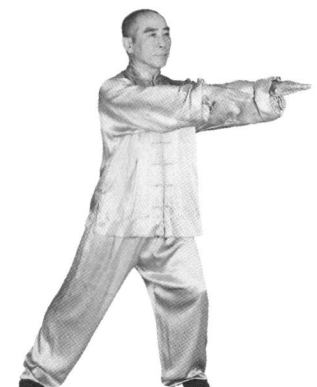

Figure 6-21

As you turn the torso 45 degrees to the right and shift the center toward the right leg, swing both arms to the right, pointing at 45 degrees. At the same time, the right hand circles down to the side of the right hip, palm facing up. Bend the left arm, crossing it in front of the chest, palm facing down, and look straight ahead (figure 6-22).

Center yourself, legs hip-width apart and slightly bent, and turn the body to the front; simultaneously, the right palm shoots upward inside the left arm and the left hand pushes downward. The left palm faces down and the right palm faces inward (figure 6-23).

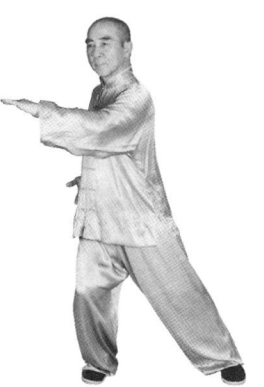

Figure 6-22

When the right palm reaches the level of the forehead and the left palm reaches the level of the abdomen, open both elbows outward and extend the right hand upward to the front right side of the head with the palm facing up. Simultaneously, push the left palm down and out to the front left side of the body, palm facing downward (figure 6-24).

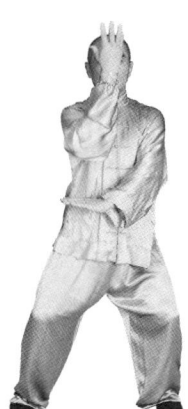

Figure 6-23

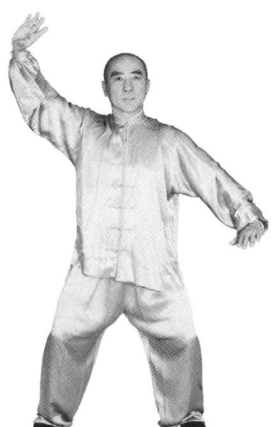

Figure 6-24

Helpful pointers: To fold is to unfold: When moving into the position in figure 6-23, slightly fold your body while keeping the body upright. Doing so provides the energy for the opening motion in figure 6-24.

To sink is to rise: When lifting the right hand up and pushing the left hand down, slightly sink the lower body to give rise to the upper body. This makes the driving energy come from the bottom of your feet.

Modification: For those who find it challenging to raise the arm above the shoulder, push the right hand forward at chest level instead.

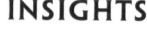

INSIGHTS

This movement originated in Chen-style Tai Chi Chuan, where it is called "Golden Rooster Stands on One Leg."

The first part of the circle brings the external force close to one's center through a circular yielding motion (figures 6-21 to 6-22); the second part of the circle applies the energy to redirect that force (figures 6-23 to 6-24). If one stopped the movement in the position illustrated in figure 6-23, the compressed energy generated through the folding process would become a constraining force, making one feel tied up, contained, restrained, or stuck. However, if one continues the flowing movement, the folding position transforms into a powerful source of expansion.

Movement 5: Flying Arrow Chases the Tiger, or Cover Hand and Thrust Fist (Figures 6-24 to 6-29)

From the position in figure 6-24, drop the right hand down and raise the left hand to shoulder height, both palms face down (figure 6-25).

Float both hands down close to the front side of the hips (figure 6-26);

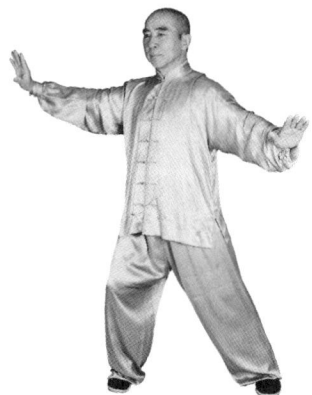

Figure 6-25

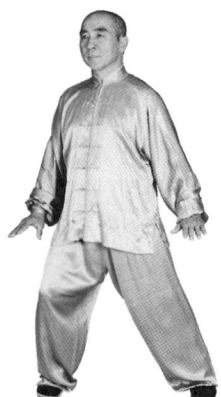

Figure 6-26

push both hands back slightly and swing them up in an outward circular movement, then bring them together in front of you into a "V" shape slightly above the shoulders, bending the elbows slightly and with the palms facing up (figure 6-27).

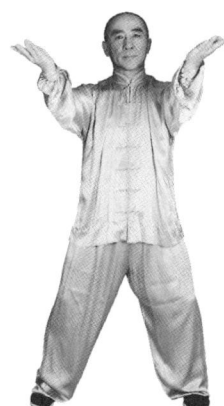

While turning the torso 45 degrees to the left, shift the center toward the left leg to form a left bow stance; simultaneously form a loose fist with the left hand facing up and draw the fist back, the end of your fist gently pressed on the belly button. At the same time, move the right arm inward slightly to the front of the center line, creating a gentle blocking energy, palm facing up and at nose height (figure 6-28).

Figure 6-27

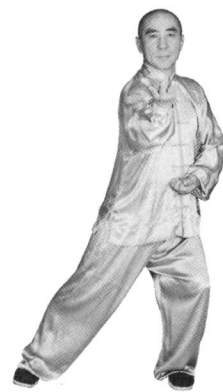
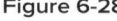

Figure 6-28

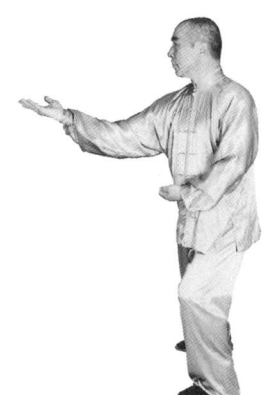

Figure 6-28B

Quickly but gently turn the torso 45 degrees to the right and shift the center toward the right leg to make a right bow stance. Pull the right palm back and make it into a loose fist to replace the left fist's position, simultaneously rolling the left fist over and punching it out over the right forearm to nose height (figure 6-29).

Helpful pointers: Modification: If raising the forearms above the shoulders is challenging, you can form the "V" shape at chest height. Keep both elbows pointing down in front of the body at a low chest height.

To sink is to engage: When throwing the left fist out, be sure to sink the body down and keep it upright, letting the energy of pulling the right hand back drive the left fist out.

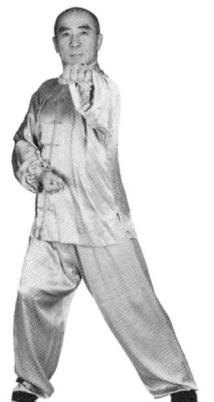

Figure 6-29

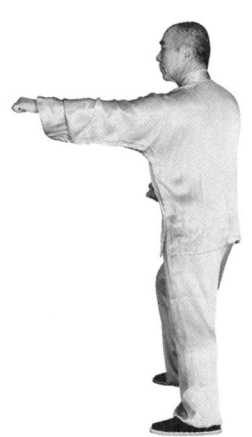

Figure 6-29B

Fly like an arrow: Avoid tensing up the left arm and fist; visualize your left fist as an arrow and the energy created by pulling your right hand back as the bow.

Have a focus: Let the arrow fly through an imagined target in front of you.

INSIGHTS

"Cover Hand and Thrust Fist" is the name for the Chen-style movement. As we discussed in the wheelchair movement 5, in the Chen style, redirecting energy can be expressed in an explosive way, like a thunderbolt in a thunderstorm. In this movement (figures 6-26 to 6-28), the motion for the first part of the circle is slow and fluid, whereas the motion for the second part of the circle is rather quick and explosive. Many practitioners enjoy this movement because it provides an experiential understanding of the power of yielding and it feels exciting.

In external martial arts, one usually punches *at* something. However, in Tai Chi Chuan, one punches *through* something. To punch through something requires calm, focused, and expanded mental space, as when one shoots an arrow from a bow. That is why this movement is called "Flying Arrow Chases the Tiger."

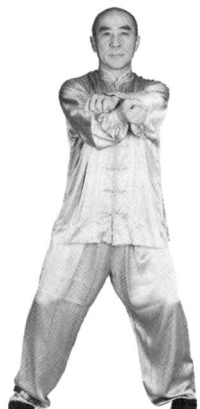

Figure 6-30

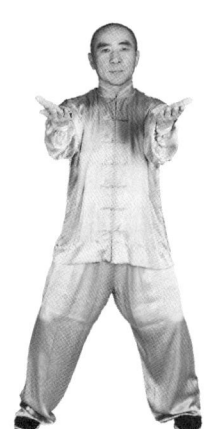

Figure 6-31

:: Movement 6: Needle at the Bottom of the Ocean (Figures 6-29 to 6-38)

From the position in figure 6-29, as your torso turns to face front, shift the body center to between the legs; slowly slide the right fist along the underside of the left forearm until the wrists cross, right fist facing up and left facing down (figure 6-30).

Slowly open the fists and turn both palms outward to shoulder height, palms facing up (figure 6-31).

Slowly bend the elbows and turn the palms so they face forward as you roll the arms back to the front of the chest (figure 6-32).

Drop the elbows down slightly and push both palms forward in a slight curving-up motion with palms facing forward and elbows slightly bent (figure 6-33).

As you turn the torso 45 degrees to the left and shift the body center to the left leg to form a bow stance, drop the left arm down and pull the left palm back to the side of the hip with the palm facing up. Simultaneously, bend your right elbow a little more and let the right palm move across the center line to the left, palm facing left and the wrist at shoulder height (figure 6-34).

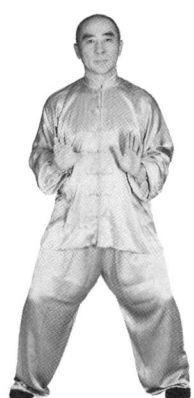

Figure 6-32

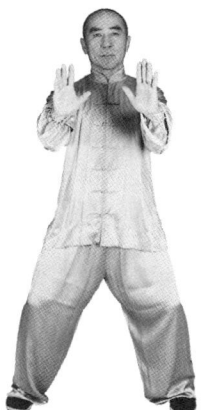

Figure 6-33

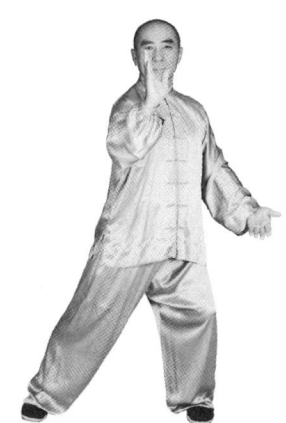

Figure 6-34

As you swing the left hand in an outward and upward curve to the front of your left shoulder with the palm facing right, the right hand continues the blocking motion downward to the position above the left knee, the palm facing up (figure 6-35).

As you turn the torso 45 degrees to the right and shift the body center to the right leg to form a right bow stance, pull the right hand across the abdomen and swing it out and upward to the right side of the body, with the palm facing up, while the left hand moves across the face to the right (figure 6-36).

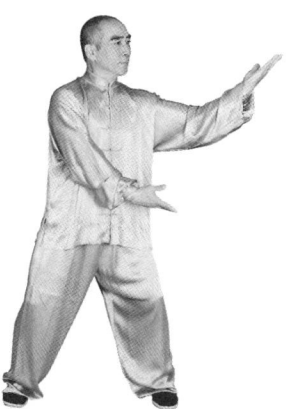

Figure 6-35

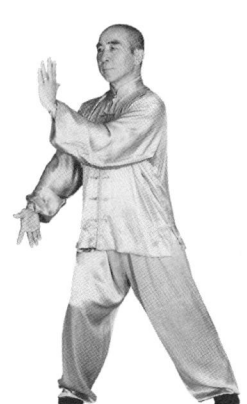

Figure 6-36

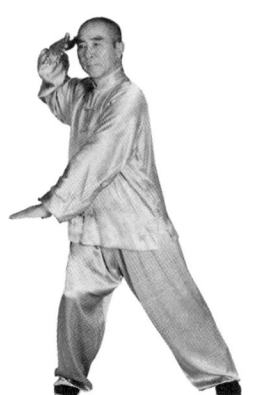
Figure 6-37

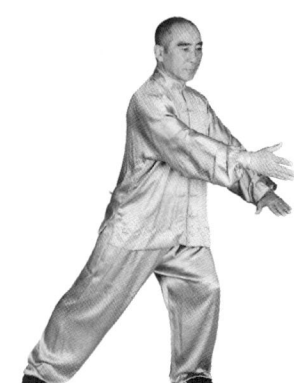
Figure 6-38

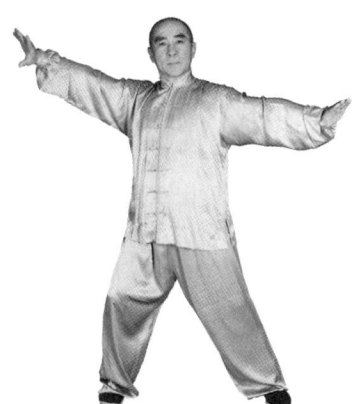
Figure 6-39

The right hand continues to float up alongside the body to pass the shoulder and arrive at the side of the head, thumb pointing up and palm facing the right temple. At the same time, the left hand circles down to the right side of the hip with fingers pointing slightly down (figure 6-37).

While turning the torso 45 degrees to the left and shifting the body center toward the left leg, move the left hand across (blocking-away energy) the body to the left side of the hip, with the palm facing down. Strike the right hand down to the left, with the thumb pointing up and fingers pointing downward 45 degrees (figure 6-38).

Helpful pointers: The revolving door effect: When moving through the two blocking motions (figures 6-33 to 6-36), the upright body turns like a revolving door.

Yin and yang: As the body turns to the left, let the left hand (yin) lead the right hand (yang), and vice versa.

Root to engage: The power that drives the striking-down movement should come from rooting the body to the ground.

Mental focus: When striking the right hand down, visualize your palm, like a spear, striking down to spear a fish at the bottom of the ocean.

INSIGHTS

The first two turning movements block or deflect an incoming force through the revolving door energy, similar to the "wax-on and wax-off" movement. The second part of the circle (figures 6-37 to 6-38) is the striking-down motion driven by the energy generated through the two blocking movements.

⦂ Movement 7: Bend the Bow to Shoot the Tiger (Figures 6-38 to 6-43)

From the position in figure 6-38, while rotating the torso 45 degrees to the right and shifting the body center to the right leg, push the left hand slightly out and swing the right arm out to the right in an up-and-down curve across the forehead, palm facing out, right hand slightly higher than the left (figure 6-39).

Both hands continue floating down to the sides of the hips. Turn your head to the left to prepare for the movement of warding off (*Peng*) (figure 6-40).

As you rotate your torso 45 degrees to the left and shift the body center toward the left leg, both arms float upward and leftward to shoulder height and width (ward-off energy). Keep the elbows slightly bent and look toward your hands (figure 6-41).

While turning the torso 45 degrees to the right and shifting the body center toward the right leg, roll the arms downward across the body to the right with palms facing down. When both hands circle up to the right side of the head, change the palms into fists, bend both elbows, and place the left fist in front of the right elbow. The heart of the right fist faces up slightly and the heart of the left fist faces right (figure 6-42).

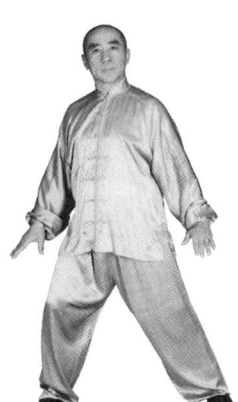
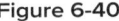

Figure 6-40

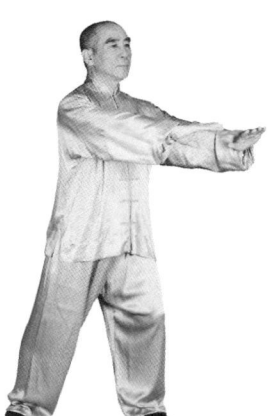

Figure 6-41

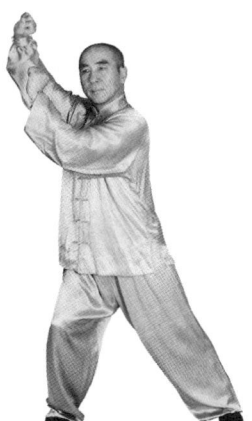

Figure 6-42

While keeping the center of the body toward the right leg, slightly turn the body to the left, simultaneously striking out both fists 45 degrees to the left. The right fist is slightly above the right forehead and the left fist is away from the body at nose height with the elbow bent (figure 6-43).

Helpful pointers: Flow like water: The rolling-down motion after the ward-off movement is flowing and circular, like a waterfall.

Stand like a tree: When turning the body to the left to strike, be sure that the energies come from the body's sinking and turning motions.

Modification: If raising the right arm above the shoulder is hard on your shoulder (figure 6-43), you can lower the right hand to any level you find comfortable.

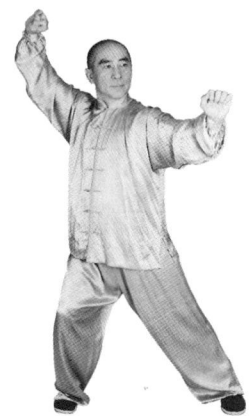

Figure 6-43

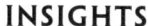

INSIGHTS

Practicing this movement evokes for me the image of bow hunters on horseback. The swing of both arms to the left is the energy of warding off, then it changes to rollback energy as you roll the hands down and across the knees to the right. Finally, the rollback motion cultivates the energy of "bend the bow to shoot the tiger."

Most important, sinking into the feet as you make the turn gives more power to the striking movement. The standing posture transforms into a dynamic power source for the movement.

Closing Form (Figures 6-43 to 6-52)

From the position in figure 6-43, rotate the body to face the front while extending the arms behind you at shoulder level, palms facing out (figure 6-44).

As the palms turn to face up, bring the arms to the front in a circular motion; both hands are shoulder width and slightly below shoulder height (figure 6-45).

Gently pull the arms back to the sides of the hips, palms facing up (figure 6-46).

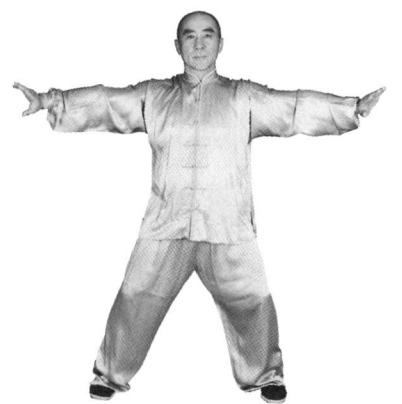

Figure 6-44

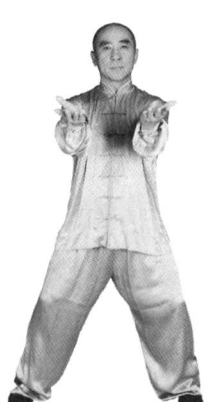

Figure 6-45

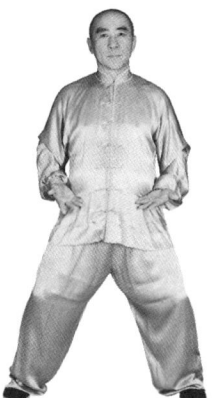

Figure 6-46

Circle your arms outward to shoulder height and turn the palms to face down (figure 6-47).

Bring both hands out and to the front; keep the arms at shoulder width and at shoulder height, palms facing down (figure 6-48).

Gently bring both hands down to the sides of the legs (figure 6-49).

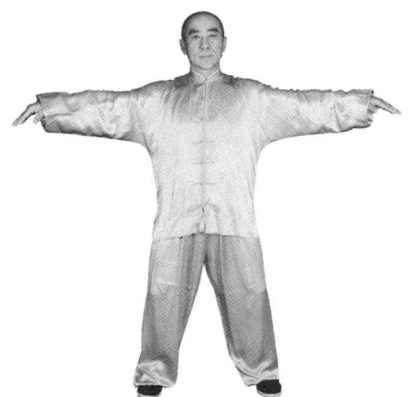

Figure 6-47

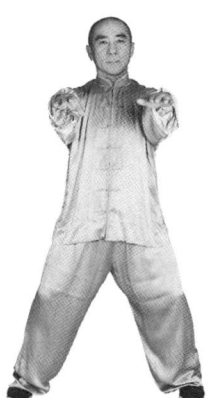

Figure 6-48

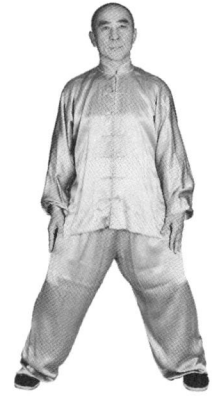

Figure 6-49

As you shift the body center to the right leg, lift the arms out from the sides, palms up. Turn the palms to face down when both hands reach the front top of the forehead. Bring the left foot close to the right and gently push the hands down to the sides of the legs (figures 6-50 to 6-52).

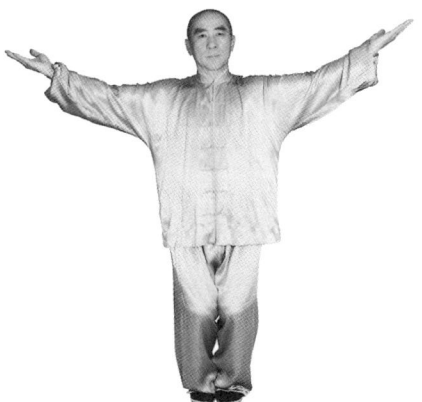

Figure 6-50

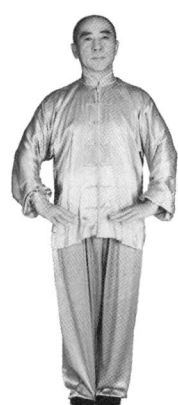

Figure 6-51

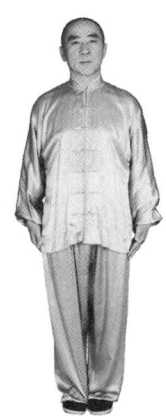

Figure 6-52

Helpful pointers: Body moves the arms: When extending the arms out at shoulder height, be sure that the arm movement synchronizes with the motion of rotating the body (figures 6-43 to 6-44).

Synchronization: When bringing both hands from the sides of the shoulder to the front, synchronize the turning of the arms and the palms to face up (figures 6-44 to 6-45).

Relax the shoulders: Avoid tensing up the shoulders when pulling the arms back and swing them out to the front through the hips (figures 6-46 to 6-48).

Modification: If raising the arms above the shoulders is challenging (figures 6-50 to 6-51), you can raise the arms up to a comfortable height— for example, to the height of the chest.

A big circle: The entire closing movement is a big circle with a few turns here and here. Making the motion flow like a gentle stream gives a sense of calm focus and closure.

Take a moment: After bringing the arms down to the sides and the left foot next to the right, stand there for a few seconds before moving on to the next activity.

THE COMMENCING AND CLOSING FORMS

See the last section of chapter 5, "The Commencing and Closing Forms," to learn about the symbolism and function of the opening and closing forms.

7

Step Like a Cat and Move Like a Wheel
Walking Tai Chi Chuan

O NE AFTERNOON some years ago, after conducting a wheelchair Tai Chi Chuan class for a group of veterans with ambulatory disabilities, a participant's spouse walked over to me and said, "My husband loves the practice so much and does it at home every day. I wish I could practice with him." It turned out that Mrs. V. had taken some Tai Chi Chuan classes at a local YMCA years before. She enjoyed these classes but had to stop attending after her husband's mobility began to decline. I asked why she had not kept up the practice at home. She said the program was long and she had forgotten most of the movements, though she had always enjoyed the group practice.

A week later I showed Mrs. V. the walking seven-posture adaptive Tai Chi Chuan program I developed to accompany the wheelchair Tai Chi modality that her husband was learning. She was delighted with the demonstration and asked me to teach her. She called me a few weeks later to say that she had just had a great practice session with her husband in their living room and they were very tickled that they were completely in sync with the movements. "It is amazing that we can practice Tai Chi together," she said joyfully.

The walking modality was developed in response to a specific need but offers broader applications. During the past seven years of implementing this modality throughout the VA healthcare system, many healthcare providers told me that it not only allowed veterans of diverse physical conditions to practice a Tai Chi program together, which promoted powerful feelings of unity, camaraderie, and inclusiveness, but also provided a practical self-care and empowering tool for practitioners. Since practicing this modality does not require much space and it takes less than three minutes to complete the sequence, many healthcare providers often practice it in their office to become fully present before starting their clinic routines or to reset during the day between rounds.

Who would benefit from this modality? The walking modality is suitable for anyone with ambulatory ability. It is an accessible and effective way of engaging and empowering the mind and body with practically no environmental constraints or space limitations.

Key features: Like the wheelchair, standing, and sitting practice modalities presented in the previous chapters, the seven-posture walking modality is an effective and convenient option for a quick Tai Chi Chuan practice session to get ready for the day, navigate a busy daily routine, or wind down from the day. The walking practice offers two unique characteristics: (1) it can be practiced anywhere with a minimum space requirement, and (2) the movements can be synchronized with the wheelchair, standing, and sitting practices, giving participants of different physical and health conditions a truly inclusive practice experience.

The walking modality also focuses on integrating each turn and step with the upper-body flowing movements and making them the driving force for the upper-body movements. Engagement with these dynamically varied and integrated movements can empower and transform our experiences of the body, mind, and space. The body that turns, steps forward, or steps backward expresses the mantra that a small step can lead to big and empowering changes.

Disclaimer: Engaging in any physical exercise can lead to injury or discomfort. These practices are not intended as medical advice or treatment and do not replace medical supervision and treatment. Please consult with your healthcare provider before starting the practice.

⁞ Preparatory Posture (Figure 7-1)

While standing, keep your knees slightly bent and let the body sink downward, keeping the head, neck, and body upright and holding the head straight up as if suspended from above by a thread. Release all tension from the shoulders and arms, letting the arms hang gently at your sides. Mentally connect all relaxed body parts to your body center (spinal cord and legs), making them a calm and engaged body system. Eyes look straight ahead, their gaze like two swords that look through everything before you.

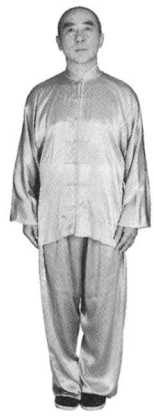

Figure 7-1

Helpful pointers: Imagine standing like a tree: bend your knees slightly and sink the lower part of your body downward like a rooted tree.

To sink is to rise: As the lower body (below the hip) is rooted into the ground like a sturdy tree trunk, raise the upper body like flourishing tree branches that give out powerful energy.

⦙ Commencement (Figures 7-2 to 7-5)

Slowly shift the body center toward the right leg, step to the left, and with the feet parallel and shoulder-width apart, open the toes slightly outward (figure 7-2).

Bend knees slightly (sinking the weight), slowly raise both arms to shoulder height, palms facing down, and relax the wrists (figure 7-3).

Without stopping, bring the arms to the front, shoulder-width apart and shoulder height with the elbows pointing down and palms relaxed and facing down (figure 7-4).

While bending your legs slowly into a comfortable position, bend and drop the elbows and draw the arms slightly inward; press your forearms down to the front of the abdomen. Keep both hands shoulder-width apart (figure 7-5).

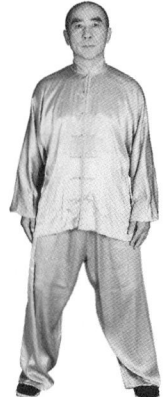

Figure 7-2

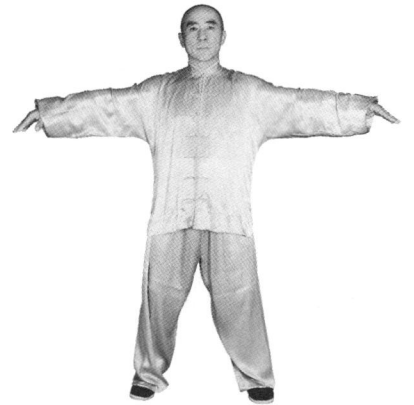

Figure 7-3

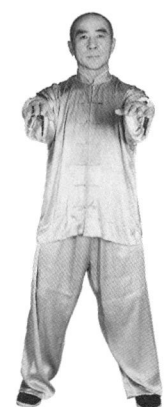

Figure 7-4

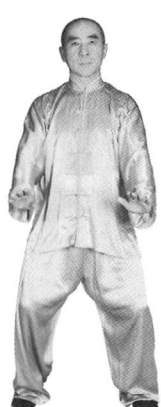

Figure 7-2

Helpful pointers: The distance between the feet for the opening stance can vary. Once the stance is set, try to stand as a rooted tree and do not move your feet during the practice.

Keeping the knees slightly bent is the key to creating a centered flow in Tai Chi Chuan practice. However, one must avoid bending the knees too deeply and moving the kneecaps freely during practice. Two practical rules of thumb: always keep the kneecaps behind the toes and face forward throughout the practice. This not only makes the practice more powerful and enjoyable, but also prevents knee discomfort.

To stand is to rise: As the arms rise slowly to reach shoulder height, keep the elbows slightly bent and pointed down; imagine that the force lifting your arms comes from the low back as your body sinks downward.

Push without pushing: When pushing your arms downward, focus on the center of the palms; visualize that you are slowly pushing a beach ball into water.

INSIGHTS

The commencement is a circular movement in two parts. The first part of the circle (figures 7-2 to 7-4) denotes the energy of yielding to or compiling the massive incoming forces (stressors) and bringing them close to your center; the second part of the circle (figures 7-4 to 7-5) denotes the energy of redirecting the compiled force downward through a flowing movement. As you push both arms down, feel the energy of your upper body rising up: rooting to rise.

Many people also like to visualize the sun rising when raising their arms and the sun setting when pushing their arms down.

⁝ Movement 1: Parting the Wild Horse's Mane (Figures 7-6 to 7-7)

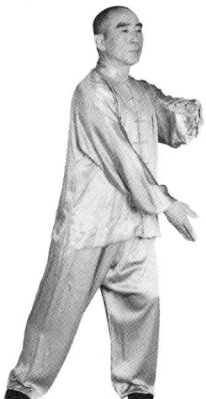

Figure 7-6

From the position in figure 7-5, shift the body center toward the left leg and slowly rotate the torso and body 45 degrees to the left to make a left bow stance. Open both arms slightly before circling the left arm to chest height and sweeping the right hand, palm facing left, across the front of your body to the left to form the "holding a ball" position under the left arm (figure 7-6).

Rotate the torso 45 degrees to the right and shift your body center toward the right leg to make a right bow stance. Slowly push the left palm down toward the side into position at the left side of the hip, simultaneously raising the right hand to chest height. Swing the right hand out 45 degrees to the right with palm facing up, ending at a position just slightly below eye level (figure 7-7).

Helpful pointers: Holding a ball: When taking the "hold a ball" position (figure 7-6), keep the left palm at shoulder height and drop the elbow, pointing down; look leftward.

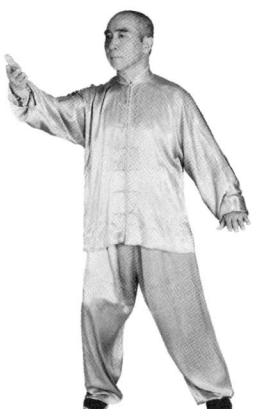

Figure 7-7

Throwing a frisbee: The movement of rotating the torso, shifting the body center from the left leg to the right, and swinging the right hand to the right is like the movement of throwing a frisbee. Let the torso do the work and the arm just follows.

Always remain centered: When you are in the motion illustrated in figures 7-6 and 7-7, be sure that your body is upright and avoid leaning the body center forward or sideways.

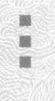

INSIGHTS

The first half of the circle for this movement (figures 7-5 to 7-6) denotes the energy of yielding to an incoming force. The process of forming the "holding the ball" position builds energy through the yielding motion. When holding the ball to the left, the torso should be slightly folded and the low-back area should feel like a gently pressed spring ready to open to the right. The second part of the circle (figures 7-6 to 7-7) denotes the energy of redirecting the incoming force through an outwardly flowing movement.

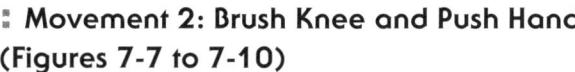

∎ Movement 2: Brush Knee and Push Hand (Figures 7-7 to 7-10)

From figure 7-7, as you rotate the torso slightly to the right, slide your right hand down with the palm facing up to the side; simultaneously, the left arm floats up to the left side of the forehead (figure 7-8).

While keeping the body center on the right leg, the right hand, with the palm facing up, swings out and upward in a circle to the side of the right ear. Turn the palm to face forward and drop the elbow; the left arm

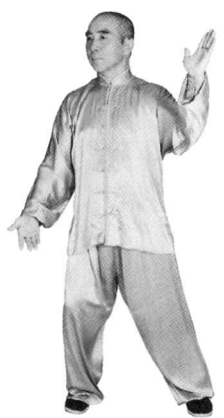

Figure 7-8

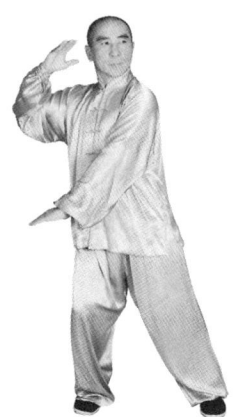

Figure 7-9

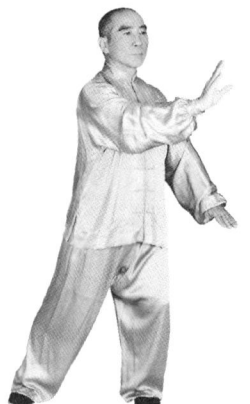

Figure 7-10

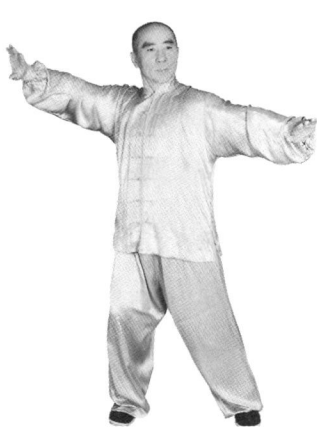

Figure 7-11

moves to cross in front of the face, passing the right shoulder to the front of the right hip (figure 7-9).

Rotate the torso 45 degrees and shift the body center to the left to make a left bow stance. Sweep the left hand downward and outward across the body to the side of the left hip with the palm facing down, and push the right hand 45 degrees to the left, with the palm facing forward and at nose height (figure 7-10).

Helpful pointers: To sink is to push: When pushing out the right palm forward (45 degrees to the left), be sure that the energy of pushing comes from sinking the body downward.

Always remain centered: When pushing (figures 7-9 and 7-10), be sure that your body is upright and avoid the body center leaning forward or sideways. Visualize pressing the body slightly backward against an invisible wall behind you for added stability.

INSIGHTS

The first half of the circle for this movement (figures 7-7 to 7-9) denotes the energy of yielding to an incoming force; the second part of the circle (figures 7-9 to 7-10) denotes the energy of redirecting the incoming force through an outward flowing movement of the body and arms.

Movement 3: Grasp the Bird's Tail (Figures 7-10 to 7-22)

Grasp the Bird's Tail is an extended and unique movement in Tai Chi Chuan. It consists of the four basic energies of engagement: expanding energy (*Peng*), rolling back energy (*Lu*), pressing or squeezing energy (*Ji*), and pushing downward energy (*An*). The instructions for these movements will also highlight the beginning and end of each of these four energies.

Ward Off with Both Arms (*Peng*) (Figures 7-10 to 7-14)

From the position in figure 7-10, rotate the torso and shift the body center to the right to make a right bow stance. Push your left hand slightly out and swing the right arm out to the right in an up-and-down curve across the forehead, palm facing out and right hand slightly higher than the left (figure 7-11).

As you slowly sink the weight down to the right foot, bend the left knee slightly and pivot on the heel 90 degrees to the left with the toe pointing to the left, then float both hands down to the sides (figure 7-12).

Continue to turn the body to the left and shift the weight onto the left leg as you put the left foot down. Bring the right foot up and take a step so it is parallel with the left foot, shoulder-width apart. Float the arms down close to the sides (figure 7-13).

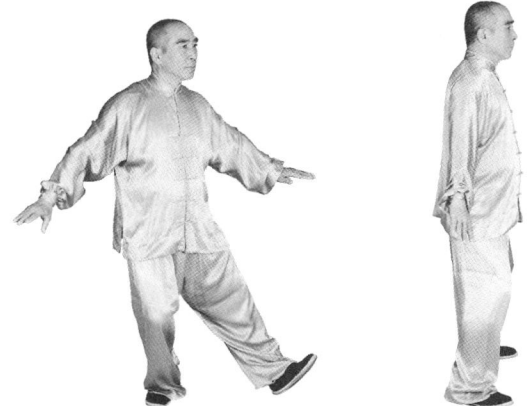

Figure 7-12   Figure 7-13

Rotate the torso 45 degrees to the left and shift the body center to the left leg. At the same time, gently lift both arms upward and leftward to shoulder height and shoulder width (ward-off energy). Keep the elbows slightly bent and pointed downward; look toward the hands (figure 7-14).

Rolling Back (*Lu*) (Figures 7-15 to 7-17)

As you lift both arms to the left and shift the body center onto the left leg completely, lift the right foot and step back behind the left to make a left bow stance. At the same time, extend the left hand forward and turn the right palm to face upward through a small circle, placing it under and touching the left wrist (figures 7-15 to 7-16).

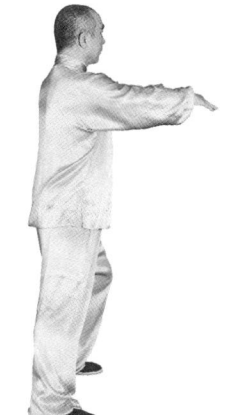

Figure 7-14

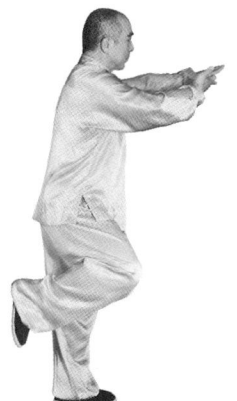

Figure 7-15

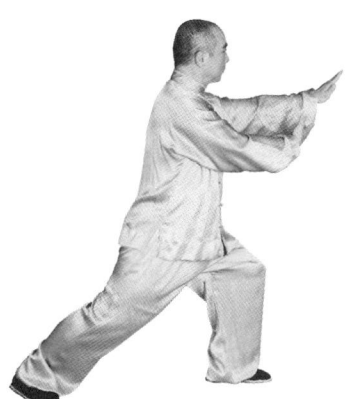

Figure 7-16

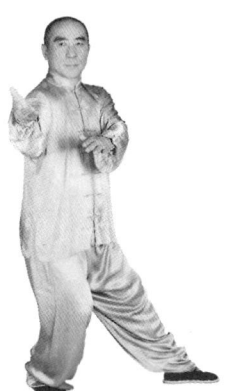

Figure 7-17

Shift the body center back toward the right leg and turn the torso 45 degrees to the right. With the left knee slightly bent and foot down, both arms roll downward and across the abdomen to the right side of your body; the eyes follow the hands (figure 7-17).

Press (*Ji*) (Figures 7-18 to 7-19)

Continue the circular motion, swinging both hands upward from the right; as the torso turns to face forward, swing both hands to the front of the chest. Place the left arm across the chest with the palm facing inward and the edge of the right hand (pinky side) against the inside of the left wrist, palm forward. Look forward and prepare to push the left hand out (figure 7-18).

As you move the torso forward into a left bow stance, the right hand presses the left inner wrist forward to form a circle at shoulder height. Keep the upper body center upright and in line with the left heel. Bend the right knee slightly. Both elbows point downward. Gaze forward (pressing energy) (figure 7-19).

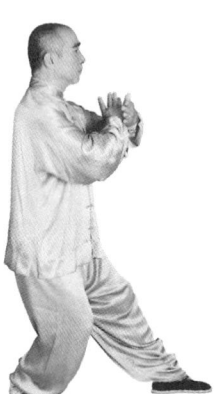

Figure 7-18

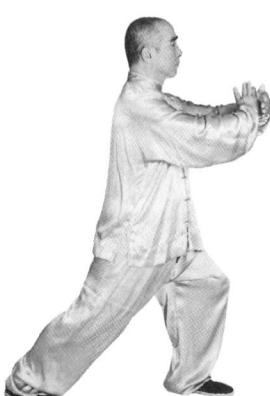

Figure 7-19

Push (*An*) (Figures 7-19 to 7-22)

Extend both hands slightly forward; the right hand crosses over the left. Turn both palms face down and open the arms to shoulder width and height (figure 7-20).

As you shift the body center back toward the right leg, drop the elbows and draw the hands back in a small up-and-down curve to the chest. The palms face down, and keep the left knee slightly bent with the toes pointing up (figure 7-21).

Without stopping, sink the body slightly downward and push the hands to the front of the abdomen. As the right foot pushes into the ground,

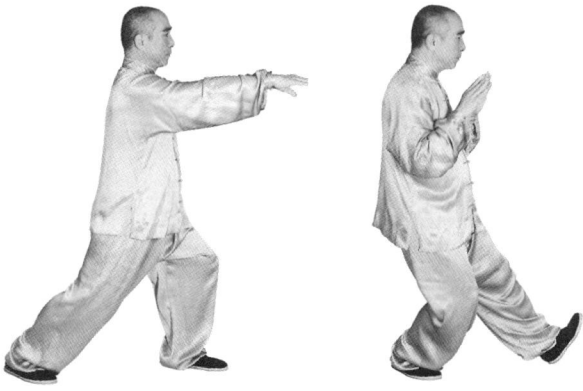

Figure 7-20   Figure 7-21

the body moves forward. Both palms turn to face forward and push with an out, up, and forward curve, at shoulder height and width (pushing energy) (figure 7-22).

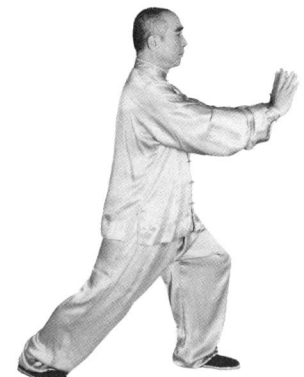

Figure 7-22

Helpful pointers: Turning like a wheel: The 90-degree left turn must be fluid, gentle, and circular, synchronizing with the movements before and immediately after. While making the turn, keep the body upright and relaxed and both knees slightly bent.

Ward off (*Peng*): The energy of lifting the arms in an upward and forward circle needs to come from envisioning the sinking of the body. Imagine that the arms are becoming connected with the feet and you use power from the rooted feet to gently ward off an oncoming force.

Rollback (*Lu*): The rollback motion should be smooth and controlled, like water flowing downhill. The rollback movement needs to be led by the turning and shifting of your body and driven by the energy of sitting back on the right leg.

Pressing (*Ji*): The energy of pressing forward should come from the actions of the body sinking and pressing back on the right leg.

Push (*An*): The movement of bringing the hands back (figures 7-18 to 7-19), bringing them down, and pushing them out (figures 7-20 to 7-22) is a wavelike circle, like redirecting an incoming force before pushing it away with another circular movement. When practicing this movement, relax the upper body, including the arms, and avoid rocking the upper body forward and backward.

INSIGHTS

Grasping the Bird's Tail is a unique movement in Tai Chi Chuan. Within one big circular movement are four smaller circles, each of which illustrates a way of engagement.

Ward off: The first half of the circle of *Peng* (figures 7-10 to 7-12) unifies or channels an external force by bringing it close to your body center through a circular movement (figures 7-12 to 7-13).

Rollback: The first half of the circle of *Lu* (figures 7-13 to 7-14) creates momentum, changes the orientation of the external force, redirects that force, and ignites the energy.

Press: The first half of the circle of *Ji* (figures 7-17 to 7-18) brings the external force close to your mind and body center and generates compressed energy between the torso and legs (figure 7-18). If movement stops there, the compressed energy will have nowhere to go and will make the body lose its balance. However, if you imagine the right leg as a compressed spring and release its energy to press the body forward, the body will press that external force away (figures 7-18 to 7-19).

Push: Like the energy of *pressing*, the *An* movements channel the incoming external force close to your center to generate the compressed energy in your torso. This energy becomes the source of power (figures 7-20 to 7-22).

These dynamic energies demonstrate how changes or challenges tend to give birth to solutions. So the great Tai Chi Chuan practitioners can use four ounces of power to move thousands of pounds as fluidly as the flowing water.

⫶ Movement 4: Golden Rooster Stands on One Leg (Figures 7-22 to 7-29)

From the position in figure 7-22, as the center of the body shifts forward onto the left leg, turn palms face down and bring the right leg up to take a step forward (figure 7-23).

As the right leg takes a small step forward and the heel lands down in front of the right shoulder with the knee slightly bent, drop the elbows slightly and let both arms move to the front of the chest in a small up-down wave (figure 7-24).

Place the entire right foot down as the body moves forward onto the right leg. Push the palms down and then move them forward as the left leg takes a small step forward so it is parallel with the right. Bend both knees slightly and keep the body upright (figure 7-25).

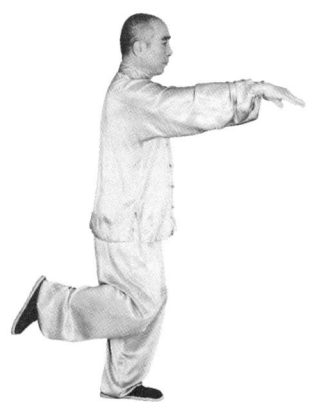

Figure 7-23

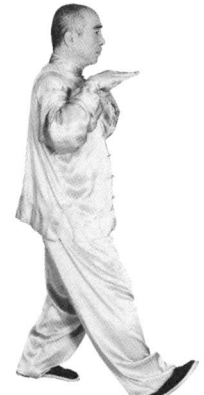

Figure 7-24

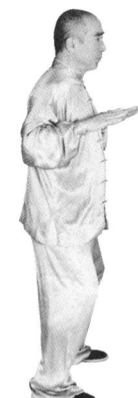

Figure 7-25

Both hands continue to push downward as they extend out in front of the shoulder as you prepare to make a right turn (figure 7-26).

As the torso turns 45 degrees to the right and shifts the body center toward the right leg, swing both arms 45 degrees to the right. The right hand continues to circle down to the side of the right hip, palm facing up, while bending the left arm, crossing it in front of the chest, palm facing down, and looking straight ahead (figure 7-27).

As the torso turns to face forward, shift the body center to the left leg; simultaneously, bring the right foot next to the left with the right toes touching the ground (figure 7-28).

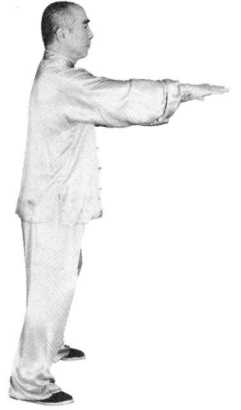

Figure 7-26

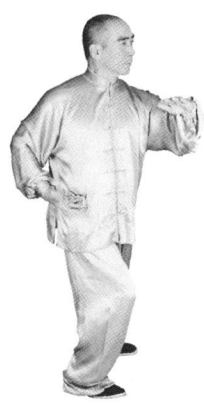

Figure 7-27

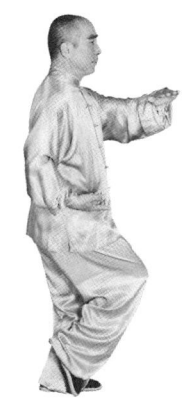

Figure 7-28

Without stopping, the right palm, facing inward, shoots upward inside the left arm while the left palm, facing down, pushes downward in a curve, bringing the right knee up along the body's center line. As the right palm reaches forehead level and the left palm reaches abdomen level, open both elbows outward to let the right hand open above and in front of the right side of your head with the palm facing up. Simultaneously, push the left palm down and out to the front-left side of the body, palm facing downward (figure 7-29).

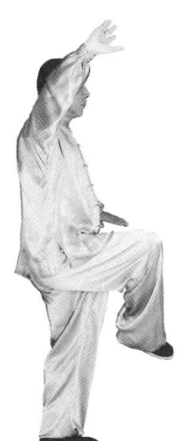

Figure 7-29

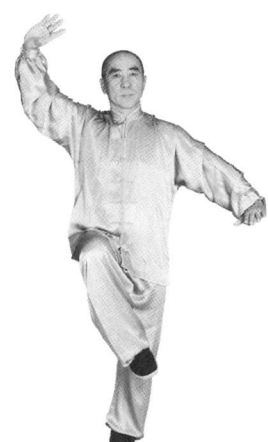

Figure 7-29B

Helpful pointers: Walk like a cat: When taking the two steps forward in figures 7-23 to 7-25, each step should be small, slow, and circular, synchronizing with the movements before and immediately after the steps. Here, lift the heel of the stepping foot first, take the step, and land with the heel first to complete the step in a curving motion.

To fold is to unfold: When moving into the position in figures 7-27 to 7-28, slightly fold your body while keeping the body upright. This will provide the energy for the opening motion in figure 7-29.

To sink is to rise: When lifting the right hand and leg and pushing the left hand down, slightly sink part of the body below the hip to give rise to the upper body. This makes the driving energy of this movement come from the bottom of the left foot.

Modification: Those who find raising the arm above the shoulder challenging could push it forward at chest level instead.

INSIGHTS

This movement originated in Chen-style Tai Chi Chuan, where it is called Golden Rooster Stands on One Leg.

The first part of the circle brings the external force close to one's center through a circular yielding motion (figures 7-26 to 7-28); the second part of the circle applies the energy generated through yielding to redirect that force (figures 7-28 7-29). If one stopped the movement in the position illustrated in figure 7-28, the compressed energy generated through the folding process would become a constraining force that makes one feel tied up, contained, restrained, or stuck. However, if one continues the movement and keeps flowing, the folding position transforms into a powerful opening motion.

The rooster is a symbol of confidence, courage, and pride in many cultures. The image of a golden rooster standing on one leg shows balance, natural beauty, and gracefulness. Therefore, mimicking this movement can also evoke those positive feelings and transform the mind and the body.

:: Movement 5: Flying Arrow Chases the Tiger, or Cover Hand and Thrust Fist (Figures 7-29 to 7-35)

From the position in figure 7-29, step down to the side with the right foot (toe lands first). At the same time, drop the right hand down and raise the left hand up to shoulder height (figure 7-30).

Shift the body center to the right leg; pivot on the left heel and rotate the torso 180 degrees to the left and swing the right leg around and step down with the left foot parallel and feet shoulder-width apart, toes pointing to the front. Bend both knees slightly and keep both arms at the sides about one foot away from the hip (figures 7-31 to 7-32).

Push both hands back slightly, swing them up in an outward circular movement, and bring them together in front of you into a "V" shape slightly above the shoulder, elbows bent and palms facing up (figure 7-33).

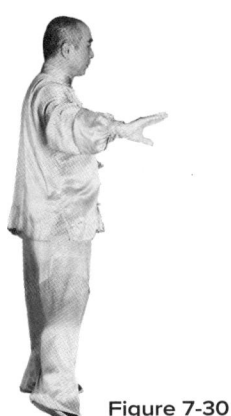 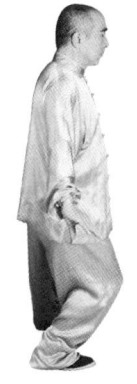 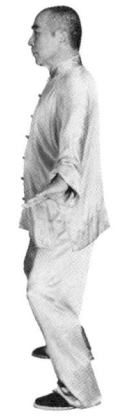 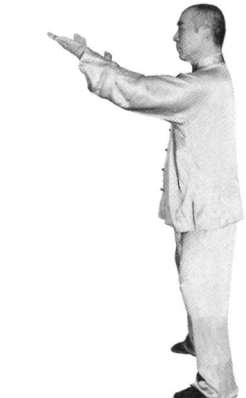

Figure 7-30	Figure 7-31	Figure 7-32	Figure 7-33

While turning the torso 45 degrees to the left, shift the body center toward the left leg to form a left bow stance. Simultaneously, make a loose fist with the left hand and draw it back: the heart of the fist faces up and the end of the fist gently presses against the belly button. At the same time, move the right arm inward slightly to the front of the center line creating a gentle blocking energy, palm facing up and at nose height (figure 7-34).

Quickly but gently turn the torso 45 degrees to the right and shift the center toward the right leg to make a right bow stance. Pull the right palm back and make it into a loose fist to replace the left fist's position,

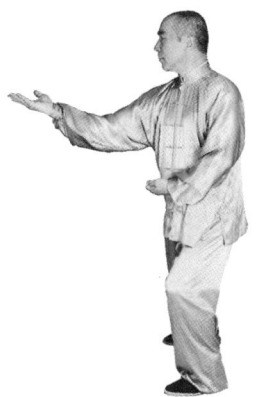

Figure 7-34

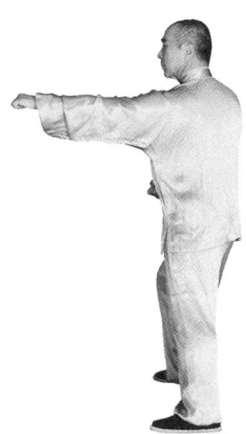

Figure 7-35

simultaneously rolling the left fist over and punching it out over the right forearm to nose height (figure 7-35).

Helpful pointers: The 180-degree turning movement needs to be slow and gentle, synchronizing with the rhythms of the upper body's movements. To make the turn flow smoothly, imagine the left heel's pivot divided into two equal parts. When landing the right foot after completing the Golden Rooster Stands on One Leg movement, shift the body center to the right leg to allow the left heel to make the first 90-degree pivoting movement (figures 7-30 to 7-31). Immediately after swinging and landing the right foot next to the left (shoulder-width apart), keep the body center slightly on the right foot to make the second half of the pivot with the left heel (figures 7-31 to 7-32). It is essential to keep the knees bent and the body upright throughout the turning movement.

Modification: If raising the forearms above the shoulder is challenging, you can form the "V" shape posture at chest height. Keep both elbows pointing down in front of the body and at low-chest height.

To sink is to engage: When throwing the left fist out, be sure to sink the body and keep it upright; this encourages you to synchronize the energies of shifting, turning, and pulling back, making these the driving force for the left punch.

Fly like an arrow: Avoid tensing up the left arm and fist; visualize your left fist as an arrow that is fired off by your body, the bow, toward an imagined target in the distance.

INSIGHTS

Cover Hand and Thrust Fist is the name for the Chen-style Tai Chi Chuan movement. As discussed elsewhere, in the Chen style, the redirecting energy can be expressed in quite an explosive way, like an arrow launched from a slowly drawn bow. The yielding energy of the first part of this circular movement slowly builds up from the end of the movement. The right-foot placement and the 180-degree turn intensifies when pulling the left hand back and crossing the right hand in front of the chest (figures 7-33 to 7-34). The second part of the circle is the punch itself: a quick release of the built-up energy.

In external martial arts, one usually punches *at* something. However, in Tai Chi Chuan, one punches *through* something. To punch through something requires calm, focus, and expansive vision, as when one shoots an arrow from a bow. That is why this movement is called "Flying Arrow Chases the Tiger."

: Movement 6: Needle at the Bottom of the Ocean
(Figures 7-35 to 7-44)

From the position in figure 7-35, after the punch, shift the weight to the right leg; as the left foot takes a small step forward, turn the torso so it faces front and slowly slide the right fist along the underside of the left forearm to cross at the wrists, right fist facing up and left facing down (figure 7-36).

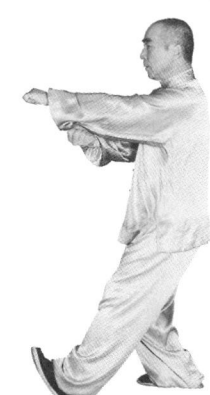

Figure 7-36

As the body center moves to the right leg to make a left bow stance, slowly open the fists and turn both palms outward at shoulder height, palms facing up (figure 7-37).

As the body center slowly moves to the left leg, make a small step forward to bring the right foot parallel with the left foot. Both feet are shoulder-width apart with toes pointing forward; at the same time, bend the elbows and turn the palms facing forward as you roll the arms inward to the front of the chest (figure 7-38).

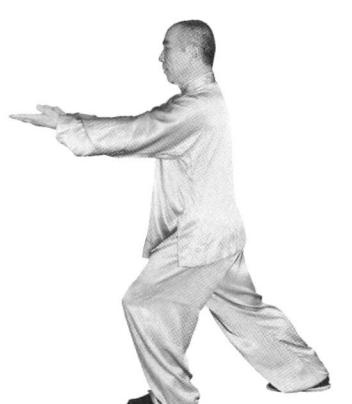

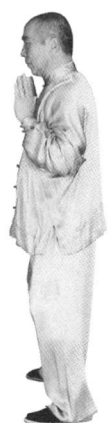

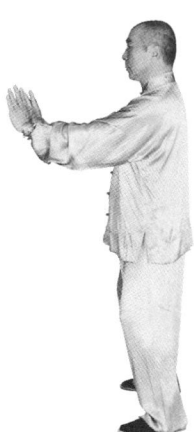

Figure 7-37   Figure 7-38   Figure 7-39

Drop the elbows down slightly and push both palms forward in a slight curving-up motion, with palms facing forward and elbows slightly bent (figure 7-39).

As you turn the torso 45 degrees to the left and shift the body center to the left leg to form a bow stance, drop the left arm down and pull the left palm back to the side of the hip with the palm facing up. Simultaneously, bend your right elbow a little more and let the right palm move across the center line to the left, palm facing left and keeping the wrist at shoulder height (figure 7-40).

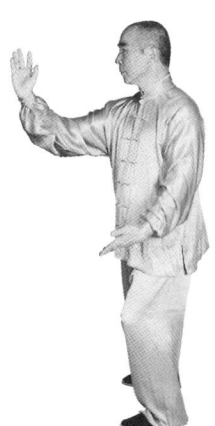

Figure 7-40

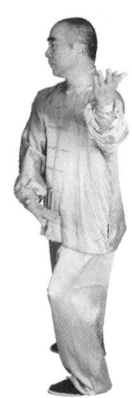

Figure 7-41

As you swing the left hand in an outward and upward curve to the front of your left shoulder with the palm facing right, the right hand continues the blocking motion down to the position in front of the left hip, with the palm facing up (figure 7-41).

As you turn the torso 45 degrees to the right and shift the body center to the right leg to form a small right bow stance, pull the right hand across the abdomen and swing it out and upward to the right side of the body, with the palm facing up, while the left hand moves across the face to the right (figure 7-42).

The right hand continues to float up at the side of the body and passes the shoulder, then arrives at the side of the head, thumb pointing up and palm facing the temple. At the same time, the left hand circles down to the right side of the hip with fingers pointing slightly down (figure 7-43).

While turning the torso 45 degrees to the left and shifting the body center toward the left leg, move the left hand across the body (blocking-away energy) to the left side of the hip, with the palm facing down. Strike down the right hand to the left, with the thumb pointing up and fingers pointing downward 45 degrees (figure 7-44).

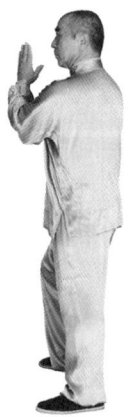

Figure 7-42

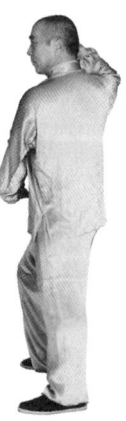

Figure 7-43

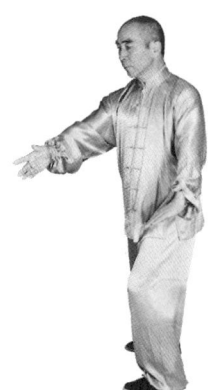

Figure 7-44

Helpful pointers: Walk like a cat: When taking the two steps forward (figures 7-35 to 7-38), each step should be small, slow, and circular, synchronizing with the movements immediately before and after the steps. Lift the heel of the stepping foot first, take the step, and land with the heel first to complete the step in a curving motion.

The revolving door effect: When moving through the two blocking motions (figures 7-39 to 7-43), keep the body upright and turn the body like a revolving door, generating energy by rotating the body center.

Yin and yang: As the body turns to the left, let the left hand (yin) lead the right hand (yang), and vice versa.

Root to engage: The power that drives the striking-down movement should come from rooting the body to the ground.

Mental focus: When striking down the right hand 45 degrees to the low left, visualize your hand, like a spear, striking down to spear a fish at the bottom of the ocean.

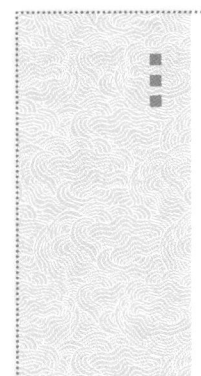

INSIGHTS

The first two turning movements block or deflect an incoming force through the body's rotation: the first part of the circle. The second part of the circle (figures 7-43 to 7-44) is the striking-down motion driven by the energy generated through the two blocking movements.

Movement 7: Bend the Bow to Shoot the Tiger (Figures 7-44 to 7-50)

From the position in figure 7-44, while rotating the torso 45 degrees to the right and shifting the body center to the right leg, push the left hand slightly out and swing out the right arm to the right in an up-and-down curve across the forehead (like the motion of opening a curtain). Right palm is facing out and the right hand is slightly higher than the left. The eyes follow the movement of the right hand (figure 7-45).

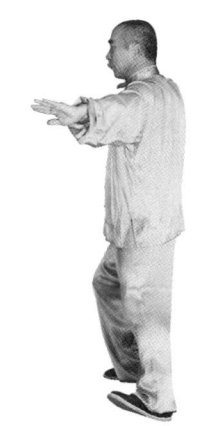

Figure 7-45

As you sink the body weight onto the right leg a little more, pivot on the left heel to turn the body 90 degrees to the left. Keep the left knee slightly bent while pivoting and point the toe forward when the turn is complete (figure 7-46).

As the body center moves to the left leg, step around with the right foot and place it parallel to the left foot and shoulder-width apart, bending both knees slightly (figure 7-47).

Bring both arms close to the thighs. As the torso turns 45 degrees to the left, shift the body center toward the left leg. Both arms float upward and leftward

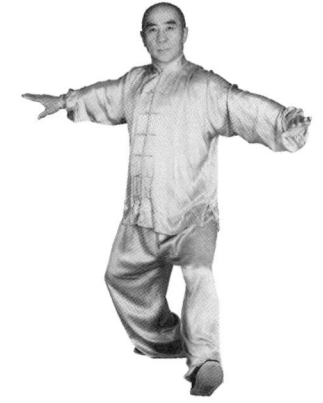

Figure 7-46

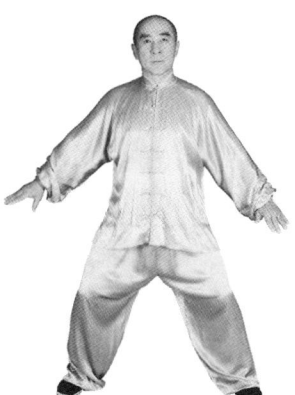

Figure 7-47

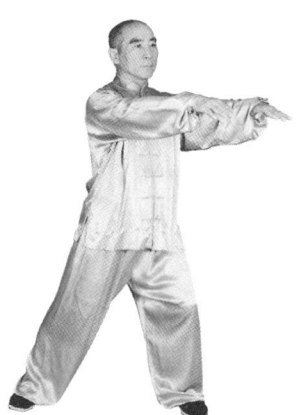

Figure 7-48

to shoulder height and width (ward-off energy). Keep the elbows slightly bent and look toward your hands (figures 7-48).

While turning the torso 45 degrees to the right and shifting the body center toward the right leg, roll the arms downward across the body to the right, with palms facing down. When both hands circle up to the right side of the head, change the palms into fists, bend both elbows, and place the left fist in front of the right elbow. The heart of the right fist faces up slightly and the heart of the left fist faces right (figure 7-49).

While keeping the body center toward the right leg, turn the body slightly to the left, simultaneously striking out both fists 45 degrees to the left. The left fist is slightly above the left forehead and the right fist is away from the body at nose height with the elbow bent (figure 7-50).

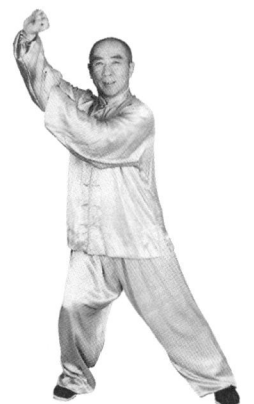

Figure 7-49

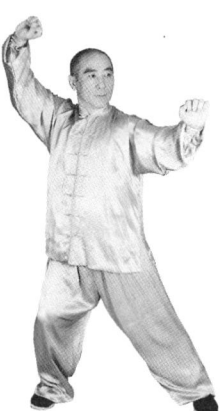

Figure 7-50

Helpful pointers: Turn like a wheel: The 90-degree turn to the left must be fluid, gentle, and circular, synchronizing with the rhythm of the movements before and immediately after the turn. While making the turn, keep the body upright and relaxed, with both knees slightly bent. Shift the body center to the left leg before swinging the right leg up gently.

Flow like water: The rolling-down motion after the ward-off movement must be flowing and circular, like a waterfall.

Stand like a tree: When turning the body to the left to strike, be sure that the energies are generated from the body's sinking and turning motions.

Modification: If raising the right arm above the shoulder is painful or uncomfortable (figure 7-49), you can lower the right hand to any level you find comfortable.

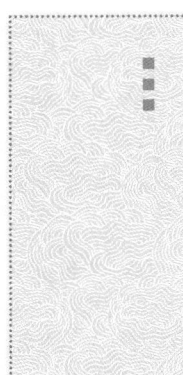

INSIGHTS

Practicing this movement always gives me the image of bow hunters on horseback. First, the swing of both arms to the left after turning the body is the energy of warding off, then it changes to rollback energy as you roll the hands down and across the knees to the right. Finally, the rollback motion cultivates the energy of "bend the bow to shoot the tiger."

Most important, sinking into the feet as you make the turn gives more power to the striking movement. The standing posture transforms into a dynamic power source for the movement.

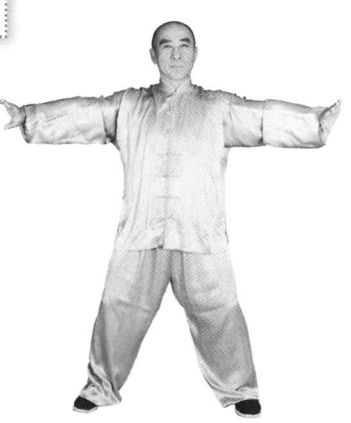

Figure 7-51

: Closing Form (Figures 7-50 to 7-59)

From the position in figure 7-50, rotate the body so it faces the front while extending the arms behind you at shoulder level, palms facing out (figure 7-51).

As palms turn to face up, bring the arms to the front in a circular motion; both hands are shoulder width and slightly below shoulder height (figure 7-52).

Gently pull the arms back to the sides of the hips, palms facing up (figure 7-53).

Circle your arms outward to shoulder height and turn the palms to face down (figure 7-54).

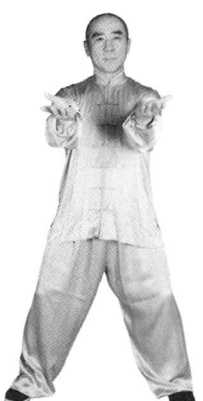

Figure 7-52

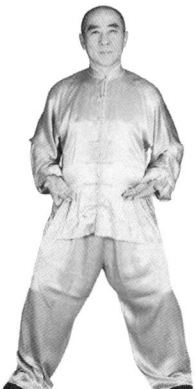

Figure 7-53

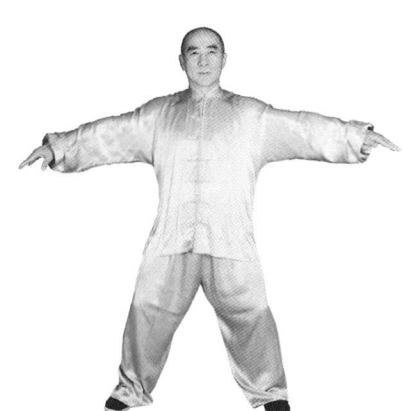

Figure 7-54

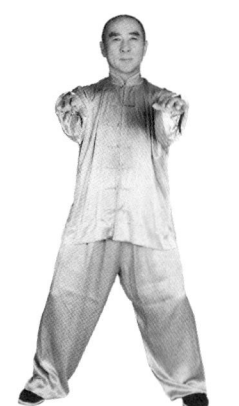

Figure 7-55

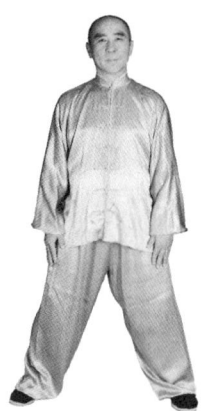

Figure 7-56

Bring both hands out and to the front; keep the arms shoulder width and at shoulder height, palms facing down (figure 7-55).

Gently bring both hands down to the sides of the legs (figure 7-56).

As you shift the body center to the right leg, lift the arms out from the sides, palms up. Turn the palms down when both hands reach the front top of the forehead; bring the left foot close to the right and gently push the hands down to the sides of the legs (figures 7-57 to 7-59).

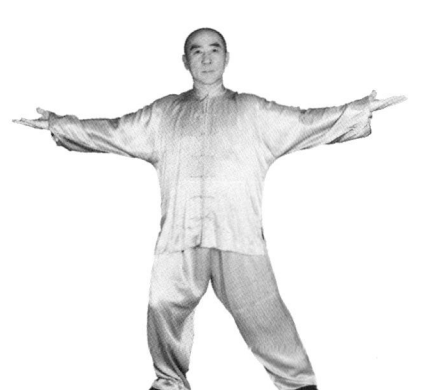

Figure 7-57

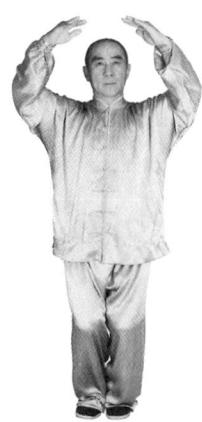

Figure 7-58

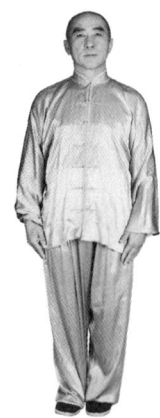

Figure 7-59

Helpful pointers: Body moves the arms: When extending the arms out to shoulder height, be sure the arm movement synchronizes with the motion of rotating the body (figures 7-50 to 7-51).

Synchronization: When bringing both hands from the sides of the shoulder to the front, synchronize the turning of the arms and the palms to face up (figures 7-51 to 7-52).

Relax the shoulders: Avoid tensing up the shoulders when pulling the arms back and swinging them out to the front (figures 7-52 to 7-55).

Modification: If raising the arms above the shoulder is challenging (figures 7-49 to 7-50 and 7-57 to 7-58), you can raise the arms up to any comfortable height—for example, to the chest.

A big circle: The entire closing movement is a big circle with a few turns here and there. Making the motion flow like a gentle stream gives a sense of calm focus and closure.

Take a moment: After bringing the arms down to the sides and the left foot next to the right, stand there for a few seconds before moving on to the next activity.

THE COMMENCING AND CLOSING FORMS

See the last section of chapter 5, "The Commencing and Closing Forms," to learn about the symbolism and function of the opening and closing forms.

8

Sit Like a Mountain and Move Like a River
Seated Tai Chi Chuan

JUST AS in a landscape the individual elements make it beautiful and powerful because they are all—mountains, flowing water, greenery, sky—different and alive, all physical conditions and all body types and postures can generate power and beauty. *Alive* can also be interpreted as *engaging*, that which transforms a quality from ordinary to extraordinary. The same can be said about our bodies and our health conditions. All physical conditions, shapes, and postures can be ordinary and extraordinary. The key is in our mind. Our mental and emotional states can transform our perceptions and engage our body to manifest physical gestures regardless of our physical condition. This perspective is part of the wisdom gleaned from nature. Therefore, sitting is a posture and can effectively engage the body and mind. The title of this chapter reflects this traditional wisdom. Contemplating the image of a grand stable mountain can harmonize the mind and emotions, and a flowing river gives rise to aliveness.

Who benefits from this modality? The seated modality of the seven-postures of adaptive Tai Chi Chuan is suitable for everyone, with or without ambulatory conditions. The practice is accessible and can effectively engage and empower the mind and body without any environmental or space limitations. One can practice this form at home or in an office or hotel room by sitting in a chair in front of a window and looking out at a tree, pond, or garden.

The features: The central idea of this modality is to make the seated position a platform for engaging the mind and creating powerful body movements that are flowing, gentle, and calming.

The chair: One can use any type of sitting device to practice. Some practitioners may want to use a chair with back support, others may want to use chairs with arms, and still others would prefer to sit on an exercise ball, depending on their body and health conditions. The most important considerations when choosing a sitting device are the following:

1. Comfortable: The sitting device allows the practitioner to sit upright with both thighs parallel to the floor and both feet on the ground, which invites a freedom of movement and promotes energy circulation during practice.

2. Strong support: The sitting device is solid and stable and can support the body and the body's movements without shifting, tipping, or wobbling.

3. The armrests: A chair without armrests makes the arm movements freer and more fluid. However, if safety is a concern, armrests help to maintain a safe body posture.

4. Back support: A chair with a back support makes the practitioner feel safer and more at ease. Many people with chronic low-back pain or similar conditions have found that practicing Tai Chi Chuan in a chair with back support allows them to freely move their torso without any pain. The practice has helped improve their back conditions.

The body: The practice of seated Tai Chi Chuan focuses on integrating the body, chair, and movements into one dynamic flow. To cultivate an empowering experience, keep the body upright but relaxed throughout the practice. Sitting like a mountain and flowing like a river is the way.

The 45-degree rotating requirement: The rotation of your body 45 degrees both left and right is an essential element of this program. The gentle, slow-flowing body rotations not only provide enormous therapeutic benefits for people with various physical and health conditions but also effectively promote the spirit of transformation and empowerment. The rotation itself becomes a source of power.

In Tai Chi Chuan, each movement must be initiated through motion in the torso or the low back. The 45-degree rotation through the torso is a reference point; the degree of the turn will depend on the physical condition of each participant. The use of gentle, circular, and a wide range of body movements during the practice offers the following benefits:

1. Reinforces the mind and body connection—for example, by focusing on the body moving the arms instead of the arms generating their own power.

2. Promotes the calming and flowing movement of the upper body.
3. Encourages circulation and a range of motion in the lower back.
4. Enhances the experience of empowerment.

Disclaimer: Engaging in any physical exercise can lead to injury or discomfort. These practices are not intended as medical advice or treatment or to replace medical supervision and treatment. Please consult with your primary healthcare provider before starting the practice.

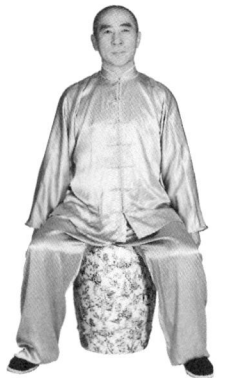

Figure 8-1

: Preparatory Posture (Figure 8-1)

While seated, keep the head, neck, and body upright, holding the head straight up as if suspended from above by a thread. Keep your shoulders relaxed and down. Release all tension from the arms and allow them to hang gently at your sides. Eyes look straight ahead, their gaze like two swords that look through everything in front of you.

Helpful pointers: Root to rise: When seated, imagine you are like a boat in the water. As your body and mind ground downward, the water (the supportive energy from the chair) lifts your body.

: Opening (Figures 8-1 to 8-4)

Slowly raise both arms to shoulder height with palms facing down. Bend the elbows and relax the wrists (figure 8-2).

Without stopping, bring the arms forward shoulder-width apart and shoulder height with the elbows pointing down, palms relaxed and facing down (figure 8-3).

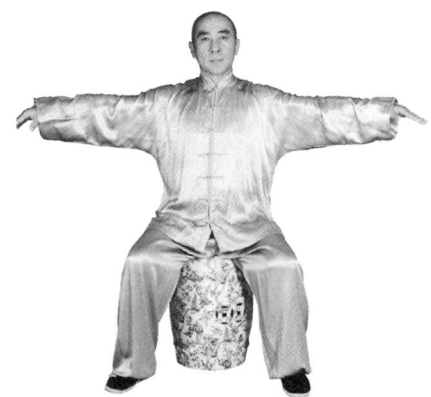

Figure 8-2

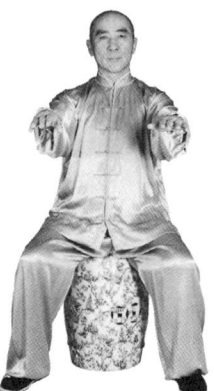

Figure 8-3

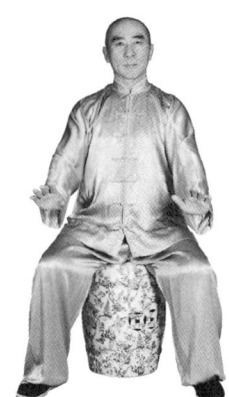

Figure 8-4

Slowly bend and drop the elbows and draw the arms slightly inward; push your forearms downward until both palms are a few inches above your knees (figure 8-4).

Helpful pointers: To sit is to rise: As the arms rise slowly to shoulder height, imagine that the force lifting your arms comes from the torso as your body sinks downward.

Push without pushing: When pushing your arms downward, focus on the center of the palms; imagine that you are slowly pushing a beach ball into the water.

INSIGHTS

The opening movement is circular, consisting of two parts. The first part of the circle (figures 8-1 to 8-3) denotes the energy of yielding to or compiling the massive incoming forces (stressors) together and bringing them close to your center; the second part of the circle (figures 8-3 to 8-4) denotes the energy of redirecting the compiled force downward through a flowing movement. As you push both arms down, feel your body rise up.

Many people like to visualize the sun rising when raising their arms and the sun setting when pushing their arms down.

Movement 1: Parting the Wild Horse's Mane (Figures 8-4 to 8-6)

From the position in figure 8-4, slowly rotate the torso 45 degrees to the left and open both arms slightly before circling the left arm to chest

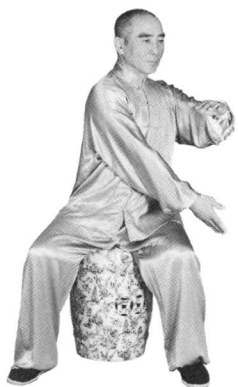

Figure 8-5

height and sweeping the right hand with palm facing left over your knees to the left, as though you area holding a big ball under the left arm (figure 8-5).

As you rotate the torso 45 degrees to the right (back to the center), slowly push the left palm down toward the outside of the left hip. Raise the right hand to chest height before swinging it out 45 degrees to the right, palm facing up, to a position just slightly below eye level (figure 8-6).

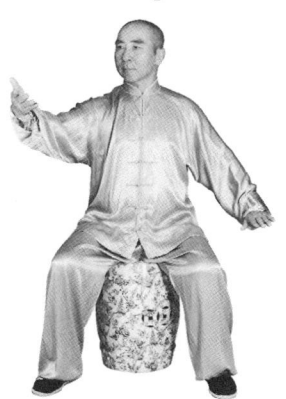

Figure 8-6

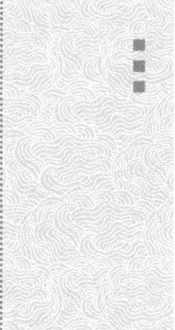

INSIGHTS

The first half of the circle for this movement (figures 8-4 to 8-5) denotes the energy of yielding to an incoming force. The process of forming the "holding the ball" position builds energy through the yielding motion. When holding the ball to the left, the torso should be slightly folded and the low-back area should feel like a gently pressed spring ready to open to the right. The second part of the circle (figures 8-5 to 8-6) denotes the built-up energy of redirecting the incoming force.

Helpful pointers: Hold a ball: When forming the "hold a ball" position, keep the left palm at shoulder height and drop the elbow down; look toward the left.

Throw a frisbee: Rotating the torso and swinging the right hand to the right is like throwing a frisbee. Let the body's rotating motion initiate the arm movements.

Stay centered: When you are in the motion illustrated in figures 8-5 and 8-6, be sure that your body is upright and avoid leaning forward or sideways.

: Movement 2: Brush Knee and Push Hand (Figures 8-6 to 8-9)

From figure 8-6, as you rotate the torso slightly to the right, slide your right hand down to the side with the palm facing up. Simultaneously, the left arm floats up to the left side of the forehead (figure 8-7).

The right hand, with the palm facing up, swings out and upward in an arc to the side of the right ear, turning the palm forward and dropping the elbow. The left arm crosses in front of the face, passing the right shoulder to arrive at the front-right side of the hip (figure 8-8).

As you rotate the torso 45 degrees to the left, sweep the left hand down-

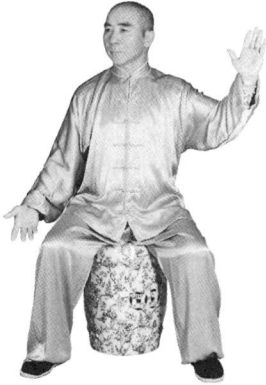

Figure 8-7

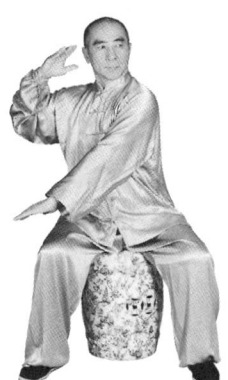

Figure 8-8

ward and outward across the front of the knees to the outside of the left knee with the palm facing down. At the same time, push the right hand 45 degrees to the left, with the palm facing forward and at nose height (figure 8-9).

Helpful pointers: The chair is the source of power: When pushing your palms forward, be sure that the power comes from the sinking of the body into the chair.

Always keep the body centered: When moving, be sure that the body is upright and avoid leaning the body forward or sideways.

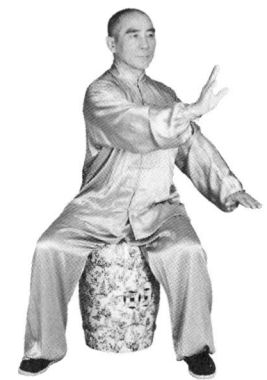

Figure 8-9

INSIGHTS

The first half of the circle for this movement (figures 8-6 to 8-8) denotes the energy of yielding to an incoming force. As you fold your torso slightly in the position illustrated in figure 8-8, the low-back area feels the energy of a gently pressed spring ready to open to the left. The second part of the circle (figures 8-8 to 8-9) denotes the energy of redirecting the incoming force through an outwardly flowing movement.

⁞ Movement 3: Grasp the Bird's Tail (Figures 8-9 to 8-19)

Grasp the Bird's Tail is a unique extended movement in Tai Chi Chuan. It consists of the four basic energies of engagement: expanding energy (*Peng*), rolling-back energy (*Lu*), pressing or squeezing energy (*Ji*), and pushing downward energy (*An*). The instructions for this movement highlight the beginning and end of each of these four energies.

Ward Off with Both Arms (*Peng*) (Figures 8-9 to 8-12)

From the position in figure 8-9, as you rotate the torso to the right, push your left hand slightly out and swing the right arm out to the right in an upward curve across the forehead, palm facing out, right hand slightly higher than the left. The eyes follow the movement of the right hand (figure 8-10).

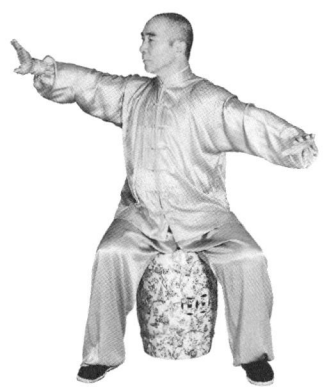

Figure 8-10

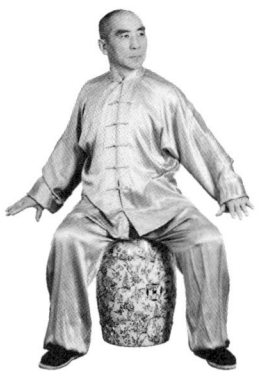

Figure 8-11

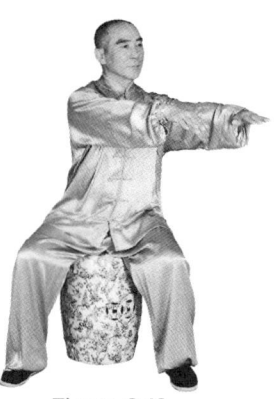

Figure 8-12

Both hands continue floating down to the sides of the hips. Turn your head to the left in preparation for the movement of warding off (*Peng*) (figure 8-11).

As you rotate your torso 45 degrees to the left, gently lift both arms upward and leftward to shoulder height and shoulder width (ward-off energy). Keep the elbows slightly bent and pointing downward. Gaze toward the hands (figure 8-12).

Rolling Back (*Lu*) (Figures 8-12 to 8-14)

From figure 8-12, as you turn the torso slightly to the left, extend the left hand forward and turn the right palm upward through a small circle, placing it at the underside of the left wrist (figure 8-13). As the torso turns 45 degree to the right, both arms roll downward and outward across the knees to the right side of the body; the gaze follows the hands (figure 8-14).

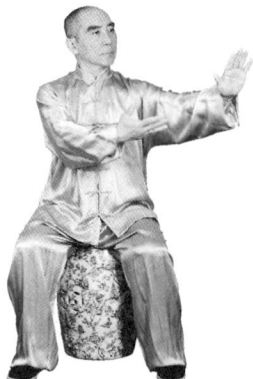

Figure 8-13

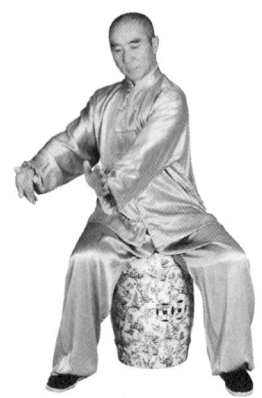

Figure 8-14

Press (*Ji*) (Figures 8-14 to 8-16)

From figure 8-14, continue the circular motion and swing both hands out and upward, passing the side of your right shoulder, and place the left arm across the chest with the palm facing the chest and the pinky edge of the right hand touching the inside of the left wrist, palm forward. Gaze forward and prepare to press the left hand outward (figure 8-15).

As the right hand presses the left inner wrist forward to form a circle at shoulder height, keep the body upright and slightly press backward; both elbows point down; gaze forward (pressing energy) (figure 8-16).

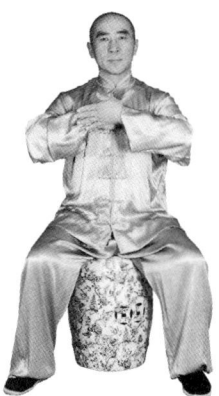

Figure 8-15

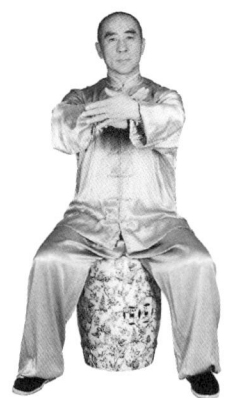

Figure 8-16

Push (An) (Figures 8-16 to 8-19)

From figure 8-16, as you extend both hands forward, the right hand crosses over the left. Turn both palms face down and open them to shoulder width and height (figure 8-17).

Bend the elbows down and draw the hands back to the front of the chest with a small curve (figure 8-18).

Without stopping, push both hands down to the front of the abdomen and then push out with an upward and forward curve, with both palms facing forward and at shoulder height and width (pushing energy) (figure 8-19).

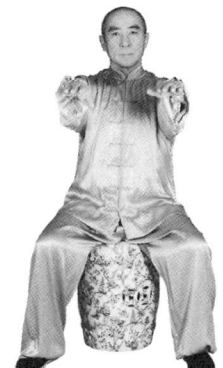

Figure 8-17

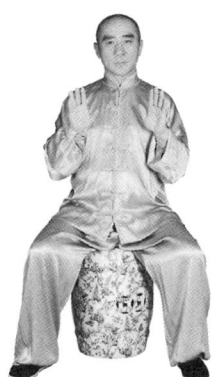

Figure 8-18

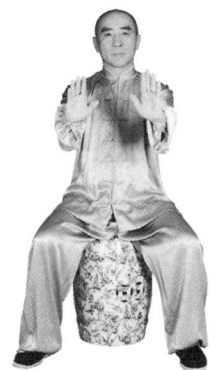

Figure 8-19

Helpful pointers: Ward off (*Peng*): The energy of lifting the arms in an arc needs to come from envisioning the sinking of the body. Imagine that the arms are connected to the feet, and you draw power from the rooted feet to gently ward off a force.

Rollback (*Lu*): The rollback motion should be smooth and controlled, like a waterfall. The rollback movement must be led by the turning and shifting of your body.

Pressing (*Ji*): The energy of pressing forward should come from the subtle movements of the body sinking and pressing back gently.

Push (*An*): The movement of bringing the hands back (figures 8-18 to 8-19), bringing them down, and pushing them out (figures 8-18 to 8-19) is circular, like redirecting a wave. When practicing this movement, relax the upper body, including the arms, and avoid rocking the upper body forward and backward.

Helpful pointers: Grasping the Bird's Tail is a unique movement in Tai

Chi Chuan. Within one big circular movement there are four smaller circles, each illustrating a way of engagement.

Ward off: The first half of the circle of *Peng* energy (figures 8-9 to 8-11) unifies or channels an external force by bringing it close to your body center through a circular movement. In doing so, it transforms and integrates the external force, which begins the second part of the circle, the ward-off movement (figures 8-11 to 8-12).

Rollback: The first half of the circle for the movement of *Lu* (figures 8-12 to 8-13) creates the momentum for the second part of the circle by changing the orientation of that external force through a small circular turn. The second part of the circle (figures 8-13 to 8-14) redirects that force through a waterfall motion using the momentum generated by the first part of the circular movement.

Press: The first half of the circle for the movement of *Ji* (figures 8-12 to 8-15) brings the external force close to your mind and body center through a circling-up movement. This yielding movement generates compressed energy between the hands and the center of the body (figure 8-15). If the movement stops there, the compressed energy will turn negative and become stuck. However, if the movement continues, the compressed energy becomes a source of power for the second part of the circle, pressing that external force away (figures 8-15 to 8-16).

Push: The first half of the circle for the movement of *An* (figures 8-17 to 8-18) channels an incoming force close to your center with an up-down curve. Like the energy of the pressing movement above, the motion of two hands rolling back generates compressed energy in your torso. This energy becomes the source of power, allowing the completion of the second part of the circle, which redirects the external force outward (figures 8-18 to 8-19).

The use of four types of energies in one circular motion implies that changes and challenges, and ways of working with them, are mutually inclusive or transformable energies. It also demonstrates how different changes or challenges tend to give birth to different solutions, and vice versa. So Tai Chi Chuan practitioners can use a force of four ounces to deflect one thousand pounds, like the flowing water.

: Movement 4: Lift the Sky and Push the Earth (Figures 8-19 to 8-23)

From the position in figure 8-19, let both palms face down. As you turn the torso 45 degrees to the left, bend your elbows slightly and turn both arms and the torso 45 degrees to the left, slightly extending the hands forward (figure 8-20).

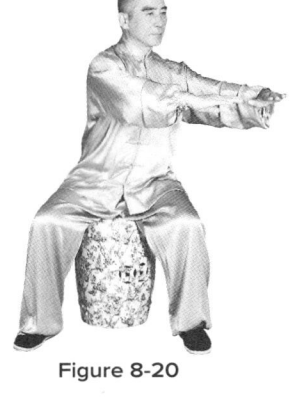

Figure 8-20

As you turn the torso 45 degrees to the right, swing both arms to the right, pointing forward. At the same time, the right hand circles down to the side of the right hip, palm facing up. Bend the left arm, crossing it in front of the chest, palm facing down, and look straight ahead (figure 8-21).

Turn the body to face front; simultaneously, the right palm shoots upward inside the left arm as you push the left hand downward, with the left palm facing down and the right facing inward (figure 8-22).

As the right palm reaches forehead height and the left palm reaches the abdomen, open both elbows outward and extend the right hand upward to the front of the right side of the head with the palm facing up. Simultaneously, push the left palm down and out to the front left side of the body, palm facing downward (figure 8-23).

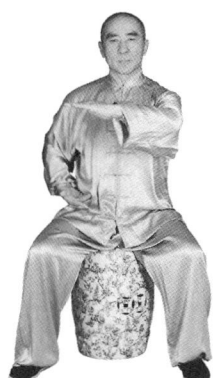

Figure 8-21

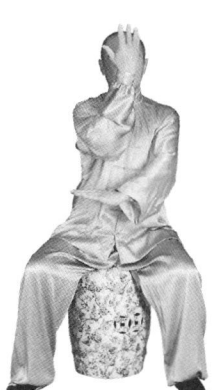

Figure 8-22

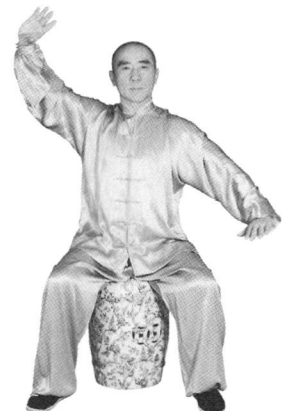

Figure 8-23

Helpful pointers: Without folding there is no unfolding: When bringing the right hand up, push the left hand down in front of the chest and try to slightly fold the torso to create compressed energy for the unfolding.

To sink is to rise: All motions—opening, unfolding, pushing down, and lifting—are driven by the energy from the body sinking down to the chair.

Sit like a mountain: Keep the body upright and avoid tensing up the shoulders, arms, and chest.

Modification: For those who find it challenging to raise the arm above the shoulder, push the right hand forward at chest height instead, or whatever is comfortable.

INSIGHTS

This movement originated in Chen-style Tai Chi Chuan, where it is called Golden Rooster Stands on One Leg.

The first part of the circle brings the incoming external force close to one's body center through a circular yielding motion (figures 8-19 to 8-21); the second part of the circle redirects that force (figures 8-21 to 8-23). Imagine if one stopped the movement in the position illustrated in figure 8-23; the compressed energy generated through folding would become a constraining force that makes one feel tied up, restrained, or stuck. However, if one continues the flowing movement, the folding position transforms into a powerful energy source.

⠇ Movement 5: Flying Arrow Chases the Tiger, or Cover Hand and Thrust Fist (Figures 8-23 to 8-28)

From the position in figure 8-23, drop the right hand down and raise the left hand to shoulder height, both palms face down (figure 8-24).

Float both hands down close to the sides of the knees (figure 8-25); push both hands back slightly and swing them up in an outward circular movement, then bring them together in front of you into a "V" shape slightly above the shoulders. The elbows are bent and palms face up (figure 8-26).

As you turn the torso 45 degrees to the left, the left hand forms a loose fist, face up and drawn back, with the end of the fist gently pressed to the belly button. At the same time, move the right arm slightly inward to the

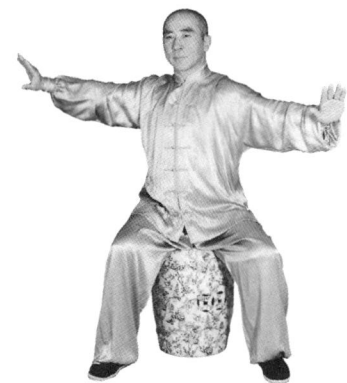

Figure 8-24

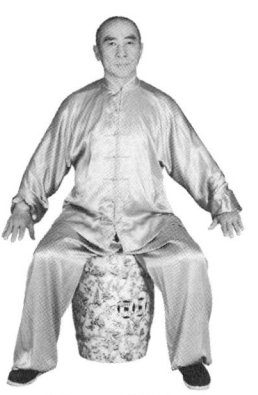
Figure 8-25

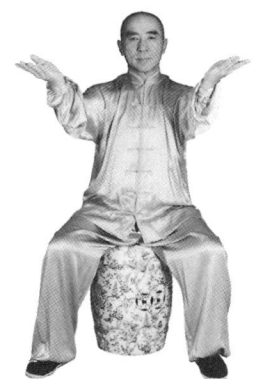
Figure 8-26

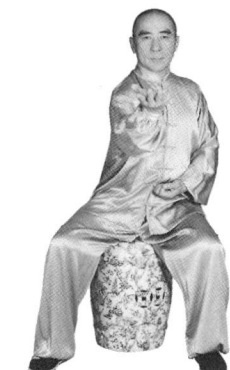
Figure 8-27

front of the center line, creating a gentle blocking energy, with the palm facing up and at nose height (figure 8-27).

As you quickly but gently turn the torso 45 degrees to the right, shift the body center toward the right leg to make a right bow stance. Pull the right palm back and change it to a loose fist to replace the left fist's position, simultaneously rolling the left fist over and punching it out over the right forearm at nose height (figure 8-28).

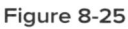
Figure 8-27B

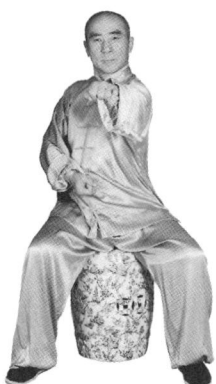
Figure 8-28

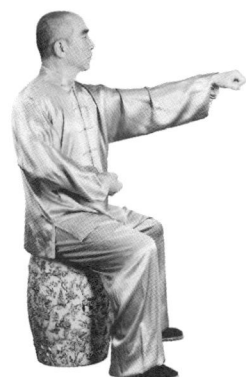
Figure 8-28B

Helpful pointers: Modification: If raising the forearms above the shoulders is painful, you can form the "V" shape at chest height. Keep both elbows pointing down in front of the body and at low chest height.

Make the chair the source of power: When throwing the left fist out, make sure to sink the body down and keep it upright, allowing the energy generated by sinking into the chair to drive the right hand back and the left fist out.

Fly like an arrow: Avoid tensing up the left arm and fist when punching; keep the fist loose and visualize your left fist as an arrow. The energy created by pulling your right hand back becomes the bow.

Have a focus: Let the arrow fly through an imaginary target before you.

INSIGHTS

Cover Hand and Thrust Fist is the name for the Chen-style movement. As we discussed in the wheelchair movement 5 and the standing movement 6, in the Chen style, redirecting energy can be expressed in quite an explosive way, like a thunderbolt in a thunderstorm. In this movement (figures 8-25 to 8-27), the motion for the first part of the circle is slow and fluid, whereas the motion for the second part of the circle is rather quick and explosive. Many practitioners enjoy this movement because it provides them with an experiential understanding of the power of yielding and it feels exciting.

In external martial arts, one usually punches *at* something. However, in Tai Chi Chuan, one punches *through* something. To punch through something requires calm, focused, and expanded mental space, as when one shoots an arrow from a bow. That is why this movement is called "Flying Arrow Chases the Tiger."

⁞ Movement 6: Needle at the Bottom of the Ocean (Figures 8-28 to 8-37)

From the position in figure 8-28, as your torso turns to face front, slowly slide the right fist along the underside of the left forearm so the wrists cross, right fist facing up and left facing down (figure 8-29).

Slowly open the fists and turn both palms outward at shoulder height, palms facing up (figure 8-30).

Slowly bend the elbows and turn the palms facing forward as you roll the arms to the front of the chest (figure 8-31).

Drop the elbows down slightly

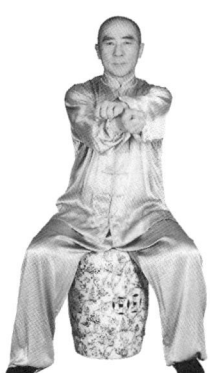

Figure 8-29

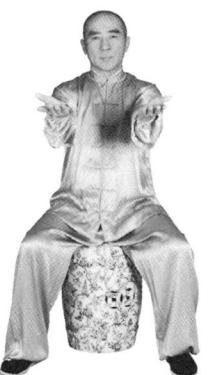

Figure 8-30

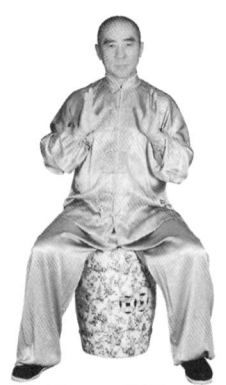

Figure 8-31

and push both palms forward in a slight curving-up motion with palms facing forward and elbows staying slightly bent (figure 8-32).

As you turn the torso 45 degrees to the left, drop the left arm down and pull the left palm back to the side of the hip with the palm facing up. Simultaneously, bend your right elbow a little more and let the right palm move across the center line to the left, palm facing left and at shoulder height (figure 8-33).

As you swing the left hand in an outward and upward curve to the front of your left shoulder with the palm facing right, the right hand continues the blocking motion downward to the position above the left knee, palm facing up (figure 8-34).

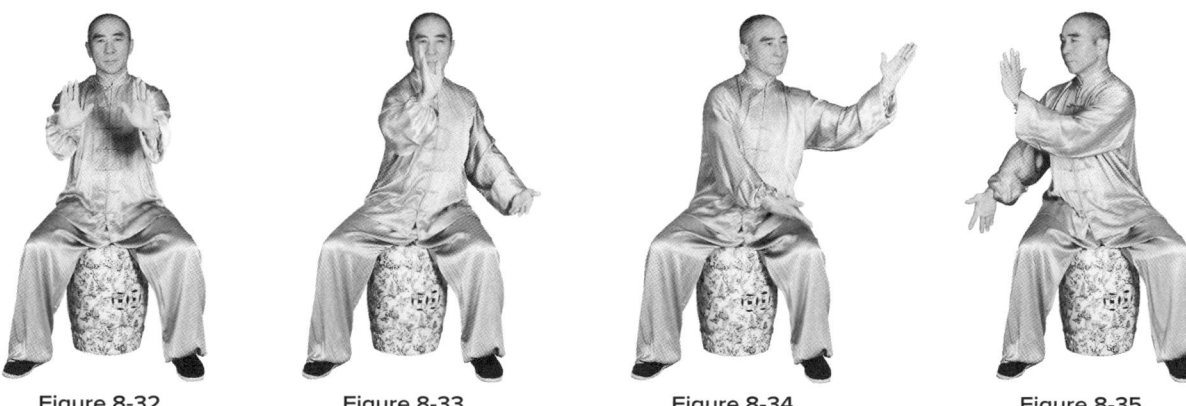

| Figure 8-32 | Figure 8-33 | Figure 8-34 | Figure 8-35 |

As the torso turns 45 degrees to the right, pull the right hand across the knees and swing the right arm out and upward to the right side of the body, palm facing up, while the left hand moves across the face to the right (figure 8-35).

The right hand continues to float up to the side of the body to pass the shoulder and arrive at the side of the head, thumb pointing up and palm facing the right temple. At the same time, the left hand circles down to the right side of the hip with fingers slightly pointing down (figure 8-36).

While turning the torso 45 degrees to the left, move the left hand across the body (blocking-away energy) to the left side of the hip with the palm facing down and strike the right hand down to the left, with the thumb pointing up and fingers pointing 45 degrees downward (figure 8-37).

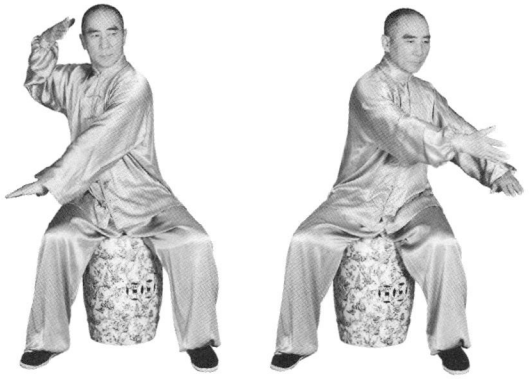

| Figure 8-36 | Figure 8-37 |

Helpful pointers: The revolving door effect: When moving through the two blocking motions (figures 8-32 to 8-35), the upright body turns like a revolving door.

Yin and yang: As the body turns to the left, let the left hand (yin) lead the right hand (yang), and vice versa.

Sit like a mountain: Keep the body upright when striking the right palm down to the left side.

Mental focus: When striking the right hand downward 45 degrees left, visualize your palm, like a spear, striking down to spear a fish.

Movement 7: Bend the Bow to Shoot the Tiger (Figures 8-37 to 8-42)

From the position in figure 8-37, while rotating the torso 45 degrees to the right, push the left hand slightly out and swing the right arm out to the right in an up-and-down curve across the forehead, palm facing out, right hand slightly higher than the left. The gaze follows the movement of the right hand (figure 8-38).

Both hands continue floating down to the sides of the hips. Turn your head to the left in preparation for the movement of warding off (*Peng*) (figure 8-39).

As you rotate your torso 45 degrees to the left, floating both arms upward and leftward to shoulder height and width (ward-off energy), keep the elbows slightly bent and gaze toward your hands (figures 8-40).

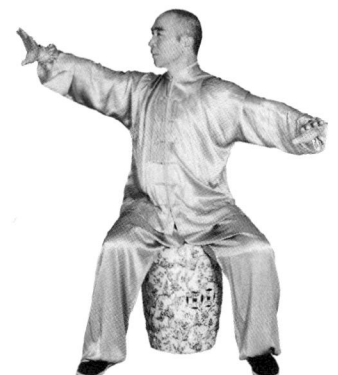

Figure 8-38

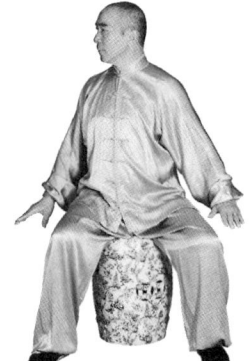

Figure 8-39

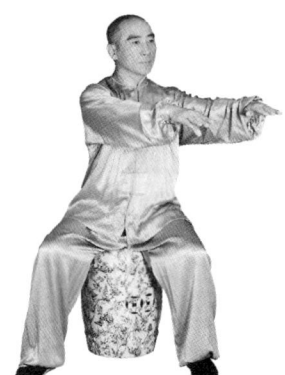

Figure 8-40

While turning the torso 45 degrees to the right, roll the arms downward across the knees to the right with palms facing down. When both hands circle up to the right side of the head, change the palms to fists, bend both elbows, and place the left fist in front of the right elbow. The heart of the right fist faces up slightly and the heart of the left fist faces right (figure 8-41).

Slightly turn the body to the left, simultaneously striking out both fists 45 degrees to the left, with the right fist positioned slightly above the right forehead and the left fist away from the body at nose height with the elbow bent (figure 8-42).

Helpful pointers: Flow like water: The rolling-down motion before the striking and after the ward-off movement is flowing and circular, like a waterfall.

Sit like a mountain: When turning the body to the left to strike, be sure that the energies come from the body's sinking into the chair and the turning motions.

Modification: If raising the right arm above the shoulder is challenging (figure 42), you can lower the right hand to any level you find comfortable.

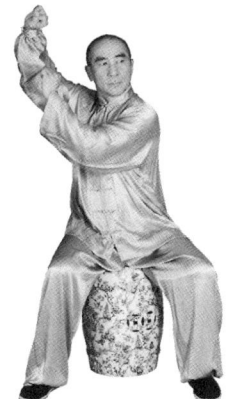

Figure 8-41

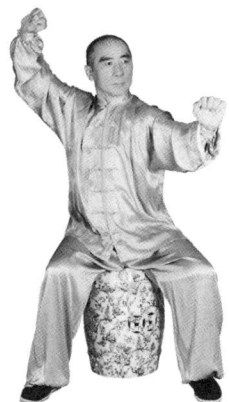

Figure 8-42

INSIGHTS

Practicing this movement evokes for me the image of bow hunters on horseback. The swing of both arms to the left after the turning of the chair is the warding-off energy, then it changes to rollback energy as you roll the hands down and across the knees to the right. Finally, the rollback motion cultivates the energy of "bend the bow to catch the tiger."

Most important, sinking into the chair and making the turn gives more power to the striking movement. The chair transforms into a dynamic power source for movement.

⫶ Closing Form (Figures 8-42 to 8-51)

From the position in figure 8-42, rotate the body to the front while extending the arms behind you at shoulder level, palms facing out (figure 8-43).

As the palms turn up, bring the arms to the front in a circular motion; both hands are shoulder width and slightly below shoulder height (figure 8-44).

Gently pull the arms back to the sides of the hips, palms facing up (figure 8-45).

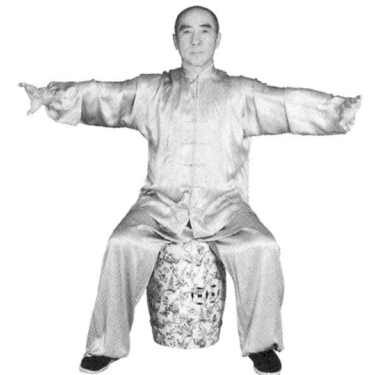

Figure 8-43

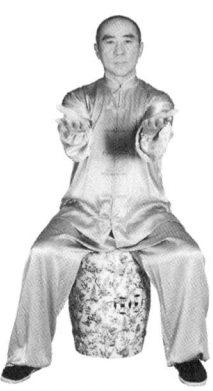

Figure 8-44

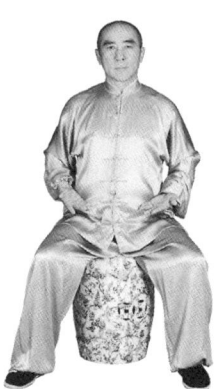

Figure 8-45

Circle your arms outward to shoulder height and turn the palms to face down (figure 8-46).

Bring both hands out and to the front; keep the arms shoulder width and at shoulder height, palms facing down (figure 8-47).

Gently bring both hands down to the sides of the legs (figure 8-48).

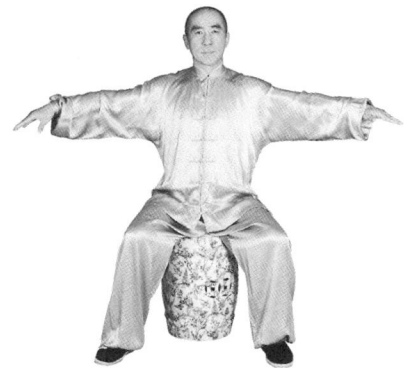

Figure 8-46

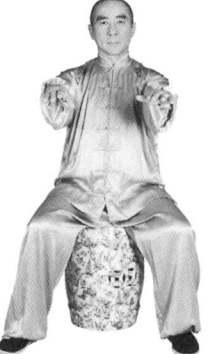

Figure 8-47

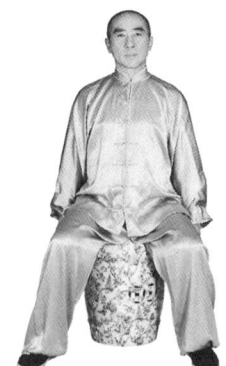

Figure 8-48

Slowly lift the arms up from the sides, palms up. Turn the palms to face down when both hands reach the front top of the forehead, and then gently push the hands down to the sides of the legs (figures 8-49 to 8-51).

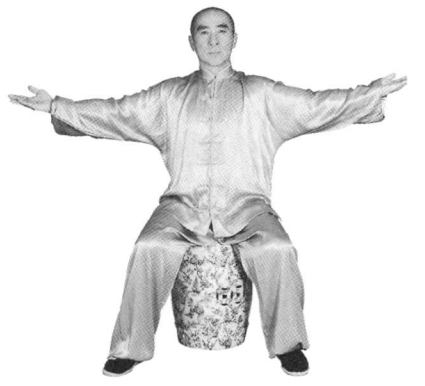

Figure 8-49

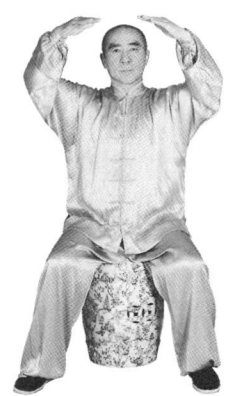

Figure 8-50

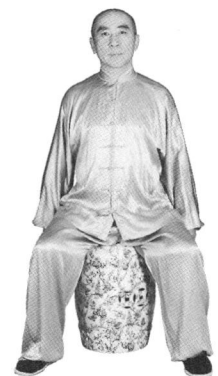

Figure 8-51

Helpful pointers: Body moves the arms: When extending the arms out at shoulder height, be sure the arm movement synchronizes with the motion of rotating the body.

Synchronization: When bringing both hands from the sides of the shoulder to the front, synchronize the turning of the arms and the palms to face up (figures 8-43 to 8-44).

Relax the shoulders: Avoid tensing up the shoulders when pulling the arms back and swinging them out to the front through the hips (figures 8-45 to 8-47).

Modification: If raising the arms above the shoulders is challenging (figure 8-50), you can raise the arms up to a comfortable height—for example, to the height of the chest.

A big circle: The entire closing movement is a big circle with a few turns here and there. Making the motion flow like a gentle stream brings a sense of calm focus and closure.

Take a moment: After bringing the arms down to the sides, sit for a few seconds before moving on to the next activity.

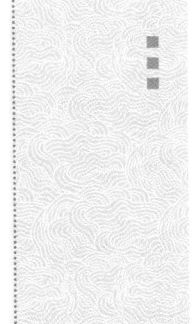

ABOUT THE COMMENCING AND CLOSING FORMS

See the last section of chapter 5, "The Commencing and Closing Forms," to learn more about the symbolism and function of the opening and closing forms.

9

One Movement, One Circle
Single-Movement Tai Chi Chuan

I WAS ONCE asked by a student, "How many movements do I have to learn to understand Tai Chi?" This is a simple question, but the answers are many and complicated. When I asked one of my teachers the same question some years ago, he told me this story.

Once upon a time, a young martial artist traveled a long way looking for a great Tai Chi master to teach him the 108 forms, the longest Tai Chi Chuan sequence. He had to master this sequence in order to fulfill his dream of one day becoming a great Tai Chi master. Eventually, he found an old master known for using wisdom to enlighten his students rather than hands-on teaching.

After the young martial artist introduced himself, the old master said: "I must farm every day. I will not have much time to teach you movement by movement. Why don't you watch me do the sequence three times, and then you can go home and practice for one year before our next lesson." The young martial artist agreed, very grateful that the old master would even consider teaching him.

One year later, the young martial artist came to see the old master. The master asked, "How many movements do you know now?" The young martial artist replied, "I remembered all 108 movements but mastered only the first sixty." The master smiled and said, "Follow me and practice the sequence three times and come to see me one year from today."

The young martial artist showed up a year later. Before the old master had a chance to ask, he said with delight, "Master, I mastered each of the 108 movements. I know exactly how each one differs from the others in practice and application." The old master smiled and said, "Why don't you follow with me to practice the movements three more times and come to see me in three years."

The young martial artist was very confused and thought, "I just told him I knew all 108 movements. Why does he still ask me to practice for three more years?" But one doesn't argue with a master. So he did as the old master asked.

The three years went by quickly. The young martial artist came to see his master. The old master looked at him and gently asked, "How many movements have you mastered now?" The young martial artist replied calmly, "One." The old master smiled and said, "You got it."

SIMPLICITY AND EFFORTLESSNESS

Only some years later when I was practicing the Tai Chi push hands (a two-person free-sparring practice) with a friend did I feel I understood a part of this story's wisdom. In college a group of us would regularly get together to practice Tai Chi Chuan and discuss philosophical ideas and their implications for modern life. Of course, the most exciting part was testing our ability to apply Tai Chi Chuan skills in friendly hand-to-hand sparring. That afternoon, I tried hard and used every move I knew to lure and redirect the force of my opponent but failed miserably. The harder I tried great or fancy moves to yield to and neutralize my opponent's force, the tighter my mind and body became. Toward the end of the practice session, I sparred with a tall, robust guy more experienced than me. Exhausted, I soon realized that my only strategic option was to hold my ground and give up the idea of pushing him away. In the middle of our exchanges, in order to yield to a force he had placed in the center of my diaphragm, I sunk my body, rotated my torso, and turned my body in a clockwise circle. The next thing I knew, he was sitting on the floor a few feet away. Both of us were shocked. I asked, "What happened? What did I do?" He replied, "I am not sure. I felt the simple circle you created, but the next thing I realized, I was in that circle." We smiled. But I still wanted to know more about his experience of being redirected by the simple circle I had created. He said, "Maybe it was because you were so tired and could not think of other fancy moves."

I learned much more from that afternoon's practice, but it's the power of simplicity that has stuck with me the most over all these years. Regardless of the number of its movements, all Tai Chi Chuan practices aim to cultivate a formless power that effortlessly deflects a challenge through one simple circular motion. This ultimate state harnesses and deploys the mind and body within just one circle. It can be achieved by practicing any number of Tai Chi movements, or just one.

SINGLE-MOVEMENT PRACTICE MODALITY BENEFITS

This chapter introduces the single-movement practice modality of the seven-posture adaptive Tai Chi Chuan program. Calling it a single-movement practice modality could be a bit misleading, as each of the seven single movements is performed on both the right and left sides and consists of two parts. In the four practice modalities introduced in earlier chapters, each movement is performed on only one side.

This single-movement modality offers many benefits:

1. *Personal preferences*: We all have favorite movements for our differently abled bodies. This modality makes it easier to practice our favorite movements and thereby meet our needs.
2. *Meditative*: This modality, especially when practiced repeatedly in one session, facilitates a calm, fluid, engaged, and meditative state of mind and body.
3. *Improved breathing*: Since the breathing can easily become rhythmic when practicing a single sequence, this modality can achieve the effects of a Qi Gong practice, which not only contributes to stress reduction, enhanced mental focus, emotional balance, and improved sleep quality but also promotes energy flow, physical well-being, and pain reduction.
4. *Symmetrical design*: Each movement is performed on both the left and right sides. Working equally on both sides promotes coordination and flexibility and builds strength throughout the body.
5. *Flexibility*: This modality is the most convenient way to practice Tai Chi Chuan. One can have a ten-minute practice session by repeatedly practicing one or more movements as time permits. If time is restricted, one can practice one movement a couple of times in even a small space. I taught this method to a physician some years ago. He still tells me how much he enjoys and benefits from the frequent practice of this modality between his morning rounds.
6. *Needs-based*: This modality can also be an ideal fitness or rehabilitation tool for folks with limited mobility due to injury. Healthcare providers from VA medical centers across the country tell me that

this modality is the most effective way to work with groups of veterans with different physical conditions. Healthcare providers can select specific movements for each person according to their needs.

7. *Accessibility*: This modality is an accessible and effective way of empowering the mind and body without special environmental or space requirements. One can practice at home or in an office or hotel room by standing before a window and looking at a tree, pond, or garden.

The illustrations of this modality show the standing posture. However, the instructions can also be applied to a sitting posture.

Each of the seven movements consists of four parts: (1) the preparatory posture, (2) the commencement form, (3) the core form, and (4) the closing form. Of course, one can add any additional core movements between a commencement and a closing form. For example, if you enjoy practicing "Lift the Sky and Push the Earth" and "Flying Arrow Chases the Tiger" together, you can start with the opening form, move through these two movements, then end with a closing form.

In chapter 6, I provided a detailed description of the standing modality, including general pointers on body posture, shifting the body center, 45-degree turning, the bow stance, the applications of the movements, and more. To avoid redundancy, the instructions for the single-movement modality focus on the sequencing of each of the seven movements.

Disclaimer: Engaging in any physical exercise can lead to injury or discomfort. These practices are not intended as medical advice or treatment or to replace medical supervision and treatment. Please consult with your primary healthcare provider before starting the training.

⠒ Movement 1: Parting the Wild Horse's Mane (Figures 9-1 to 9-14)

Preparatory Posture (Figure 9-1)

While standing, keep your knees slightly bent and sink the body downward. Keep the head, neck, and body upright, holding the head straight up as if suspended from above by a thread. Release all tension from the shoulders and arms, letting the arms hang gently at your sides. Mentally

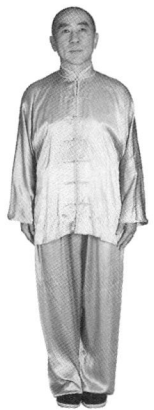

Figure 9-1

connect all relaxed body parts to your body center (spine and legs), making them a calmly engaged body system. Eyes look straight ahead, their gaze like two swords that look through everything in front of you.

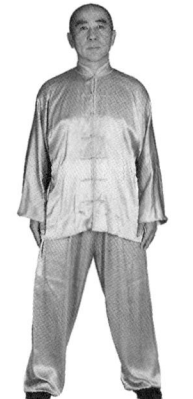

Figure 9-2

Commencing Form (Figures 9-2 to 9-5)

Slowly shift the body center toward the right leg and step to the left, keeping the feet parallel and shoulder-width apart, pointing the toes slightly outward (figure 9-2).

Slowly raise both arms to shoulder height, palms facing down, and relax the wrists (figure 9-3).

Without stopping, bring the arms to the front, shoulder-width apart and shoulder height with the elbows down, palms relaxed and facing down (figure 9-4).

While bending your legs slowly into a comfortable position, bend and drop the elbows and draw the arms slightly inward. Push your forearms down to the abdomen. Keep both hands shoulder-width apart (figure 9-5).

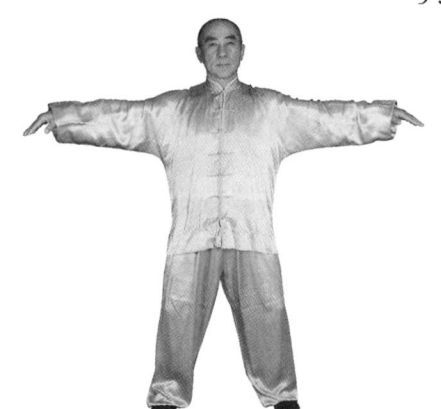

Figure 9-3

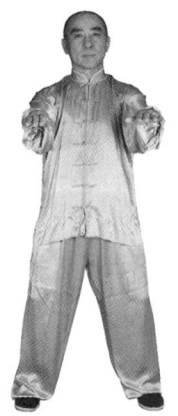

Figure 9-4

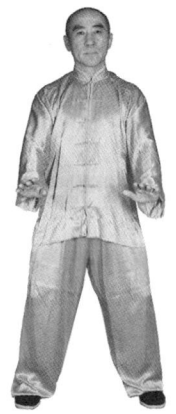

Figure 9-5

Core Form (Figures 9-6 to 9-9)

Right Side (Figures 9-6 to 9-7)

From the position in figure 9-5, shift the body center toward the left leg and slowly rotate the torso and the body 45 degrees to the left to make a left bow stance. Open both arms slightly before circling the left arm to chest height and sweeping the right hand with palm facing left across the front of your body to the left to form a "holding a ball" position under the left arm (figure 9-6).

As you rotate the torso 45 degrees to the right and shift your body center toward the right leg to make a right bow stance, slowly push the left palm down toward the side and into position at the left side of the hip. At the same time, raise the right hand to chest height before swinging it out 45 degrees to the right with the palm facing up. Position the right hand just slightly below eye level (figure 9-7).

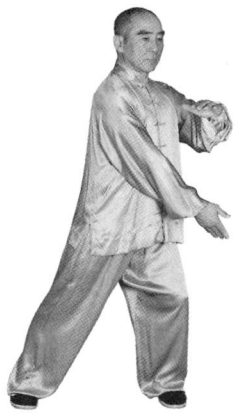

Figure 9-6

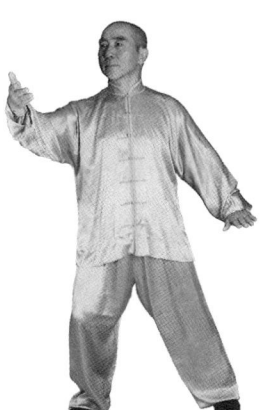

Figure 9-7

Left side (Figures 9-8 to 9-9)

From figure 9-7, slowly turn the right palm face down as the left arm floats across the diaphragm into position under the right palm, forming a ball-holding position (figure 9-8).

As you rotate the torso 45 degrees to the left and shift your body center toward the left leg to make a left bow stance, slowly push the right palm down toward the side and into position at the right side of the hip. At the same time, raise the left hand to chest height before swinging it out 45 degrees to the left with the palm slightly facing up. Position the left hand just slightly below eye level (figure 9-9).

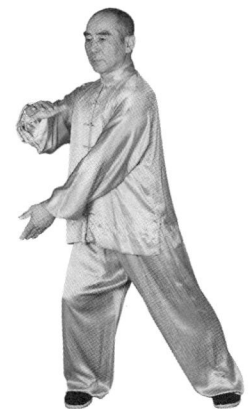

Figure 9-8

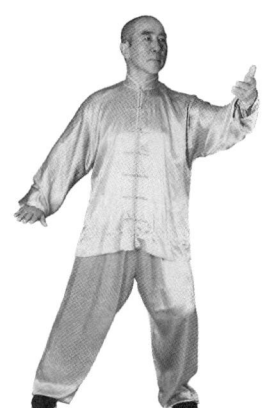

Figure 9-9

Closing Form (Figures 9-10 to 9-15)

From the position in figure 9-9, rotate the body to face the front while extending the arms behind you at shoulder level, palms facing down (figure 9-10).

Bring the arms to the front in a circular motion; both hands are shoulder-width apart and slightly below shoulder height (figure 9-11).

Gently drop the arms to the sides of the hips, palms facing the hips (figure 9-12).

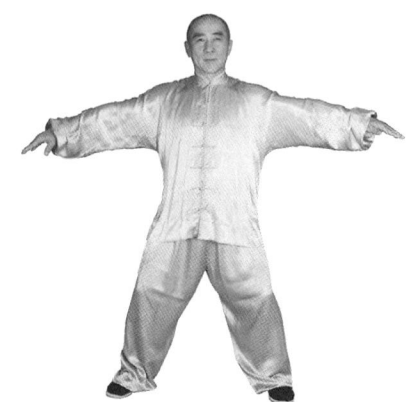

Figure 9-10

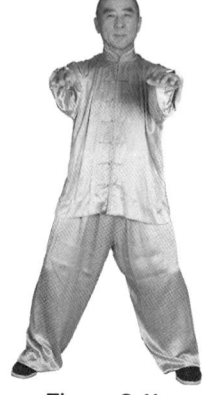

Figure 9-11

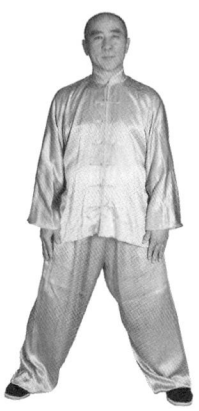

Figure 9-12

Circle your arms to shoulder height with the palms facing up. While shifting the body center to the right leg, step the left foot next to the right (figure 9-13).

Bring both palms to the front of the chest in a curved motion. Turn the palms face down and gently push both hands down from the front side of the body to rest at the sides of the body (figures 9-14 to 9-15).

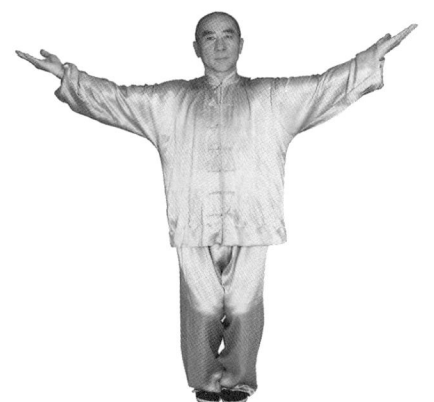
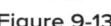

Figure 9-13

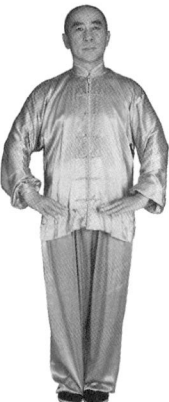

Figure 9-14

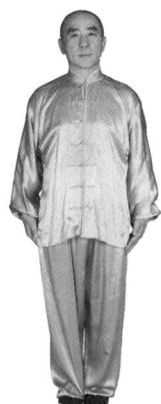

Figure 9-15

⦂ Movement 2: Brush Knee and Push Hand (Figures 9-15 to 9-30)

Preparatory Posture (Figure 9-15)

While standing, keep your knees slightly bent and sink the body downward. Keep the head, neck, and body upright, holding the head straight up as if suspended from above by a thread. Release all tension from the shoulders and arms, letting the arms hang gently at your sides. Mentally connect all relaxed body parts to your body center (spinal cord and two legs), making them a calmly engaged body system. Eyes look straight ahead, their gaze like two swords that look through everything before you.

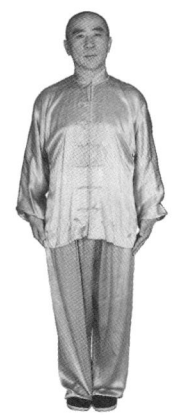

Figure 9-15

Commencing Form (Figures 9-16 to 9-19)

Slowly shift the body center toward the right leg, step to the left, and keep the feet parallel and shoulder-width apart, opening both toes slightly outward (figure 9-16).

Slowly raise both arms to shoulder height, the palms facing down, and relax the wrists (figure 9-17).

Without stopping, bring the arms to the front, shoulder-width apart and shoulder height, with the elbows down and the palms relaxed and facing down (figure 9-18).

While bending your legs slowly into a comfortable position, bend and drop the elbows and draw the arms slightly inward; push your forearms down to the abdomen, keeping both hands shoulder-width apart (figure 9-19).

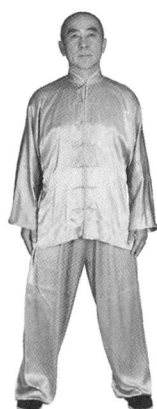

Figure 9-16

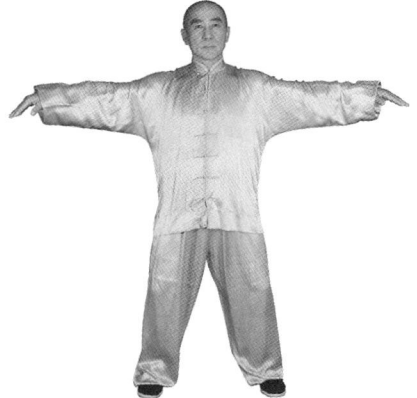

Figure 9-17

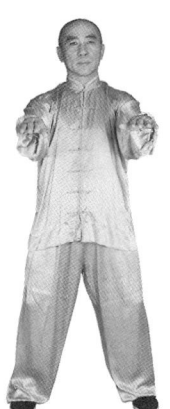

Figure 9-18

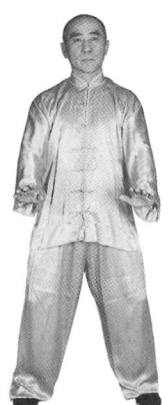

Figure 9-19

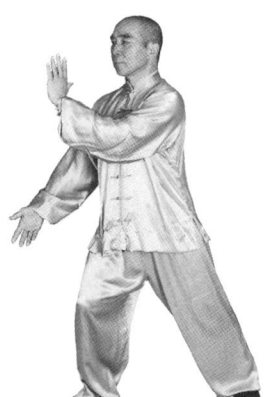

Figure 9-20

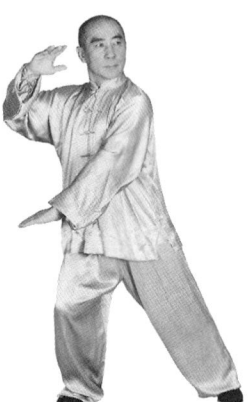

Figure 9-21

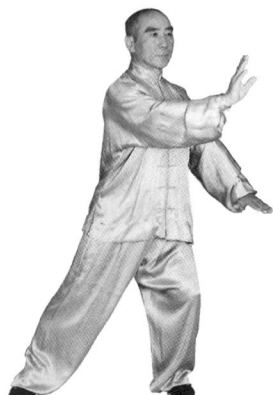

Figure 9-22

Core Form (Figures 9-20 to 9-24)

Left Side (Figures 9-20 to 9-22)

From figure 9-19, as you rotate the torso slightly to the right, slide your right hand down with the palm facing up to the side. At the same time, the left arm floats up to the left side of the forehead (figure 9-20).

While keeping the body center on the right leg, the right hand, palm facing up, swings out and up in a circle to the side of the right ear. Turn the palm to face forward and drop the elbow. The left arm crosses in front of the face, passing the right shoulder to the front-right side of the hip (figure 9-21).

As you rotate the torso 45 degrees and shift the body center to the left to make a left bow stance, sweep the left hand downward and outward across the body to the side of the left hip, palm facing down. Push the right hand 45 degrees to the left, palm forward and at nose height (figure 9-22).

Right Side (Figures 9-22 to 9-24)

Gently push the right palm down to the outer right hip and bring the left hand up to the right ear, palm facing down and forward (figure 9-23).

As you rotate the torso 45 degrees and shift the body center to the right to make a right bow stance, sweep the right hand downward and outward across the body to the side of the right hip, palm facing down. Push the left hand 45 degrees to the right, palm forward and at nose height (figure 9-24).

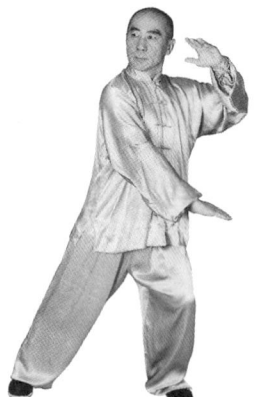

Figure 9-23

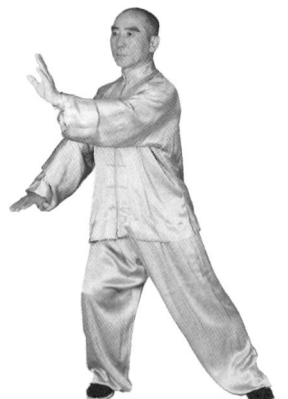

Figure 9-24

Closing Form (Figures 9-25 to 9-30)

From the position in figure 9-24, rotate the body to face the front and swing the left hand to the left. Extend the arms behind you at shoulder level, palms facing down (figure 9-25).

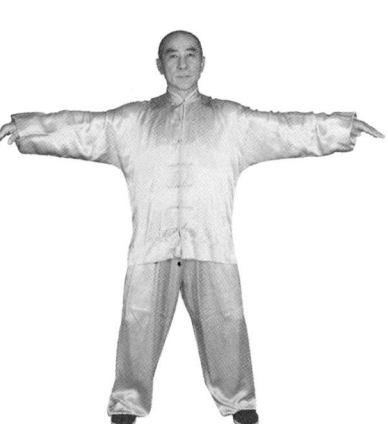

Figure 9-25

Bring the arms to the front in a circular motion; both hands are shoulder-width apart and slightly below shoulder height (figure 9-26).

Gently drop the arms to the sides of the hips, palms facing the hips (figure 9-27).

Circle your arms to shoulder height with palms facing up. While shifting the body center to the right leg, bring the left foot next to the right foot (figure 9-28).

Bring both palms to the front of the chest in a curved motion. Turn the palms face down; gently push both hands down from the front of the body to rest at the sides (figures 9-29 to 9-30).

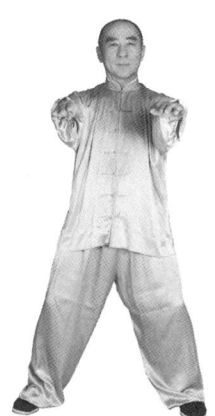

Figure 9-26

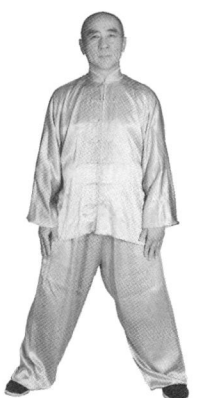

Figure 9-27

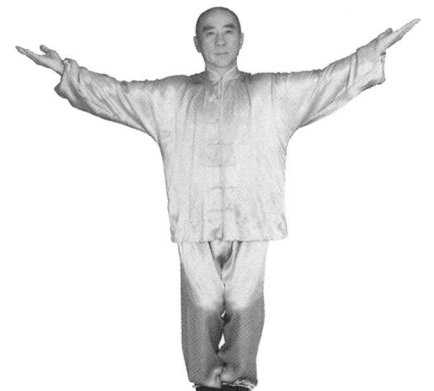

Figure 9-28

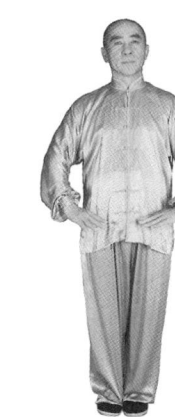

Figure 9-29

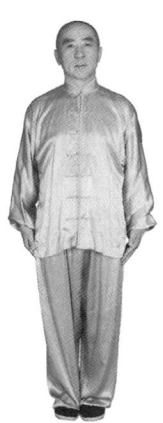

Figure 9-30

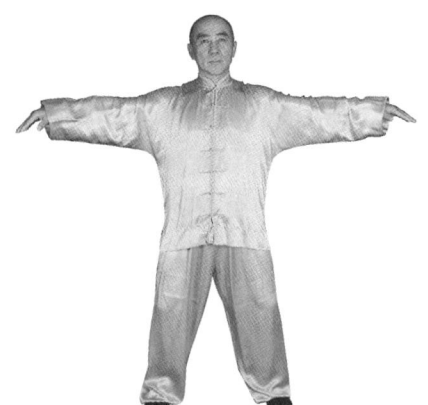

Figure 9-30

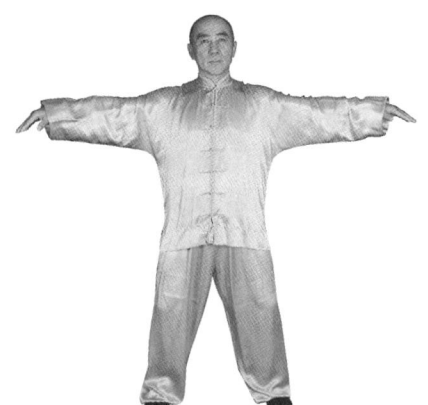

Figure 9-31

⦂ Movement 3: Grasp the Bird's Tail (Figures 9-30 to 9-56)

Preparatory Posture (Figure 9-30)

While standing, keep your knees slightly bent and sink the body downward. Keep the head, neck, and body upright, holding the head straight up as if suspended from above by a thread. Release all tension from the shoulders and arms, letting the arms hang gently at your sides. Mentally connect all relaxed body parts to your body center (spine and legs), making them a calmly engaged body system. Eyes look straight ahead, their gaze like two swords that look through everything before you.

Commencing Form (Figures 9-31 to 9-34)

Slowly shift the body center toward the right leg, step to the left, and keep the feet parallel and shoulder-width apart, opening both toes slightly outward (figure 9-31).

Slowly raise both arms to shoulder height, palms facing down, and relax the wrists (figure 9-32).

Without stopping, bring the arms to the front, shoulder-width apart and shoulder height with the elbows down, palms relaxed and facing down (figure 9-33).

While bending your legs slowly into a comfortable position, bend and drop the elbows and draw the arms slightly inward. Push your forearms down to the front of the abdomen, keeping both hands shoulder-width apart (figure 9-34).

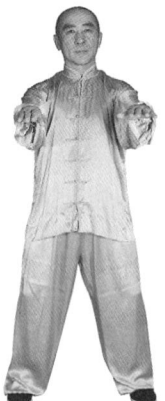

Figure 9-32

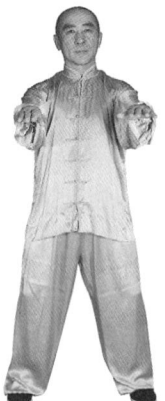

Figure 9-33

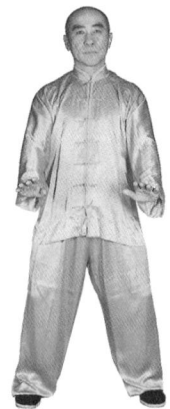

Figure 9-34

Core Form (Figures 9-34 to 9-52)

Left Side (Figures 9-34 to 9-43)

Turn the torso slightly to the left and swing both arms through a small arc 45 degrees to the left, palms facing down (figure 9-35).

Extend the left hand forward and turn the right palm to face upward, placing it at the underside of the left wrist (figure 9-36).

As you turn the body 45 degrees to the right, shift your body center to the right leg, making a right bow stance. Both arms roll downward and outward across the abdomen to the right side of your body, your gaze following the hands (figure 9-37).

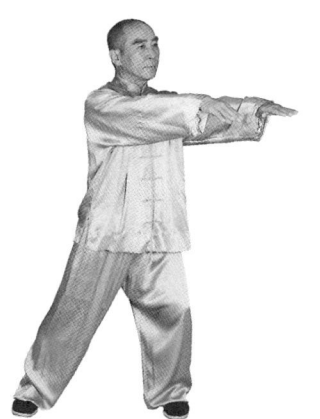

Figure 9-35

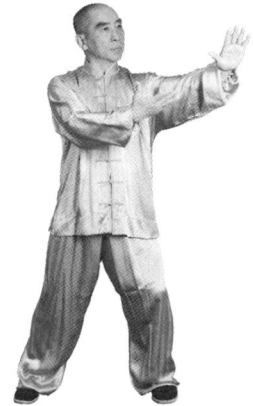

Figure 9-36

Continue the circular motion to swing both hands out and upward, passing the side of your right shoulder, and place the left arm across the chest. The palm faces the chest and the edge of the right hand (pinky side) touches the inside of the left wrist, palm forward. Look forward and prepare to push the left hand out (figure 9-38).

As the right hand presses the left inner wrist forward to form a circle at shoulder height, keep the upper body upright and press backward. Both elbows point down and the gaze is forward (pressing energy) (figure 9-39).

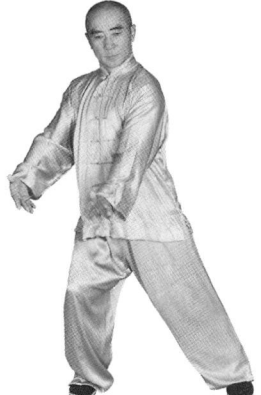

Figure 9-37

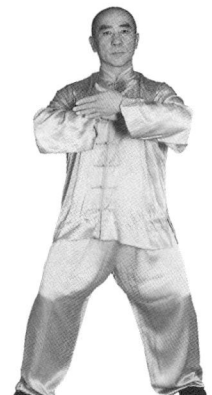

Figure 9-38

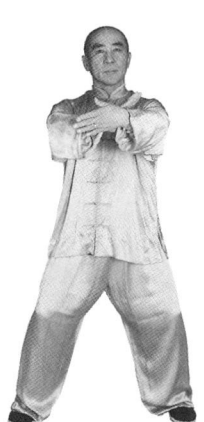

Figure 9-39

As you extend both hands forward, the right hand crosses over the left. Turn both palms face down and open them to shoulder width and height (figure 9-40).

Bend the elbows down and draw the hands back in an up-and-down curve to the chest (figure 9-41).

Without stopping, push both hands down to the front of the abdomen (figure 9-42) and then push out with an upward curve, both palms facing forward and at shoulder height and width (pushing energy) (figure 9-43).

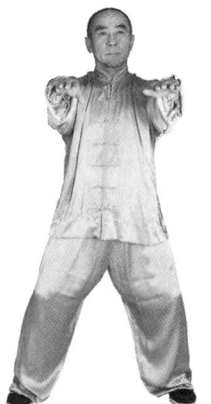 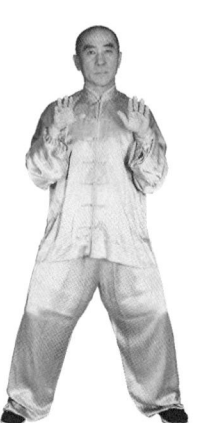 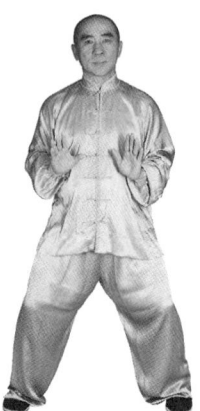 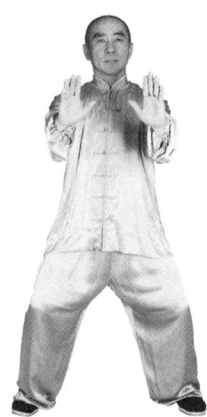

| Figure 9-40 | Figure 9-41 | Figure 9-42 | Figure 9-43 |

Right Side (Figures 9-43 to 9-52)

From the position in figure 9-43, swing both arms through a small arc 45 degrees to the right, palms facing down (figure 9-44).

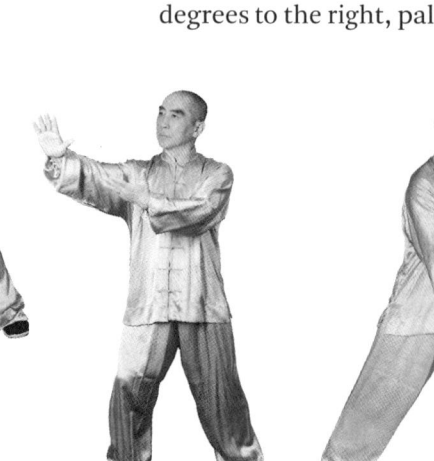 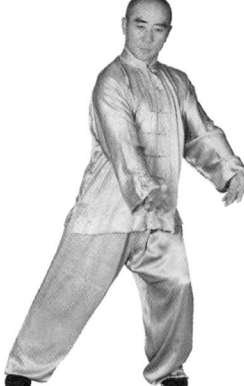

Figure 9-44

Figure 9-45   Figure 9-46

Turn the torso slightly to the right, extend the right hand forward, and turn the left palm to face upward through a small circle, placing it at the underside of the right wrist (figure 9-45).

As you turn the body 45 degrees to the left, shift your center to the left leg, making a left bow stance. Both arms roll downward and outward across the abdomen to the left side of the body, the gaze following the hands (figure 9-46).

Continue the circular motion to swing both hands out and upward, passing the side of your left shoulder, and place the right arm across the chest. The palm faces the chest and the edge of the left hand (pinky side) touches the inside of the right wrist, palm forward. Look forward and prepare to push the right hand out (figure 9-47).

As the left hand presses the right inner wrist forward to form a circle at shoulder height, keep the upper body upright and pressed backward and both elbows pointed down. The gaze is forward (figure 9-48).

As you extend both hands forward, open them to shoulder and width height, the left hand crossing over the right, both palms facing down (figure 9-49).

Bend the elbows down and draw the hands back in an up-and-down curve to the chest (figure 9-50). Without stopping, push both hands down to the front of the abdomen (figure 9-51). Then, push palms out with an upward and forward curve, both palms facing forward and at shoulder height and width (figures 9-52).

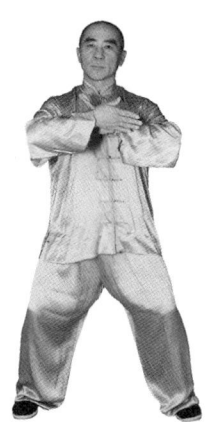

Figure 9-47

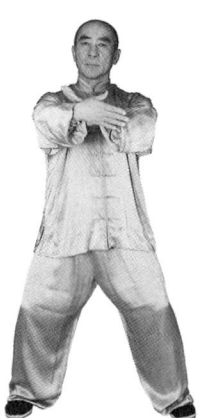

Figure 9-48

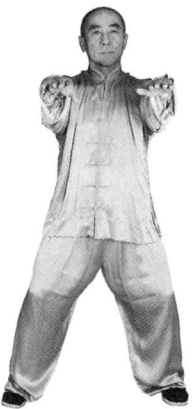

Figure 9-49

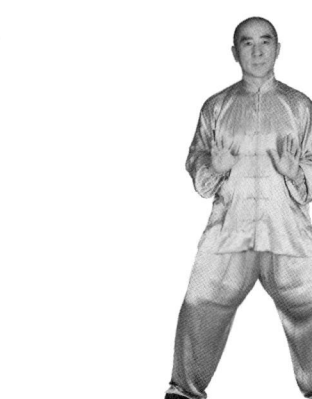

Figure 9-50

Figure 9-51

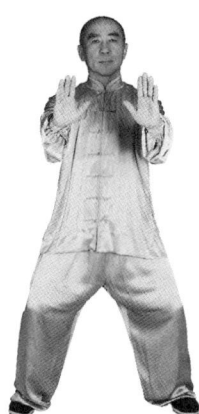

Figure 9-52

Closing Form (Figures 9-52 to 9-56)

From the position in figure 9-52, gently drop the arms to the sides of the hips, palms facing the hips (figure 9-53).

Circle your arms to shoulder height with palms facing up. While shifting the body center to the right leg, bring the left foot next to the right foot (figure 9-54).

Bring both palms to the front of the chest with a curved motion, the palms facing down. Gently push both hands down from the front side of the body and bring them to rest at your side (figures 9-55 to 9-56).

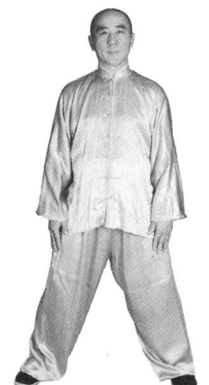

Figure 9-53

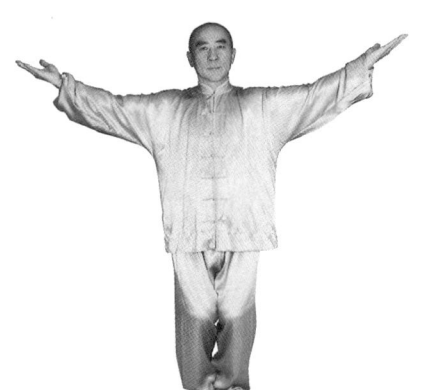

Figure 9-54

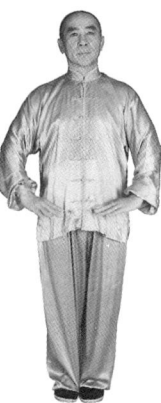

Figure 9-55

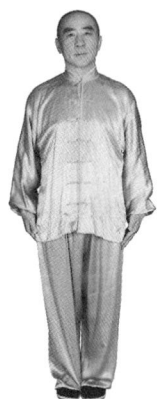

Figure 9-56

: Movement 4: Hold the Sky and Push the Earth (Figures 9-56 to 9-74)

Preparatory Posture (Figure 9-56)

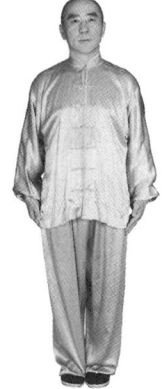

Figure 9-56

While standing, keep your knees slightly bent and sink the body downward, keeping the head, neck, and body upright and holding the head straight up as if suspended from above by a thread. Release all tension from the shoulders and arms, letting the hands hang gently at your sides. Mentally connect all relaxed body parts to your body center (spinal cord and two legs), making them a calmly engaged body system. Eyes look straight ahead, their gaze like two swords that look through everything before you.

Commencing Form (Figures 9-57 to 9-61)

Slowly shift the body center toward the right leg and step to the left, keeping the feet parallel and shoulder-width apart, opening both toes slightly outward (figure 9-57).

Slowly raise both arms to shoulder height, palms facing down, and relax the wrists (figure 9-58).

Without stopping, bring the arms to the front, shoulder-width apart and shoulder height, with the elbows down and the palms relaxed and facing down (figure 9-59).

While bending your legs slowly into a comfortable position, bend and drop the elbows and draw the arms slightly inward, pushing your forearms down to the abdomen and keeping both hands shoulder-width apart (figure 9-60).

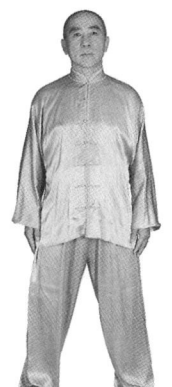

Figure 9-57

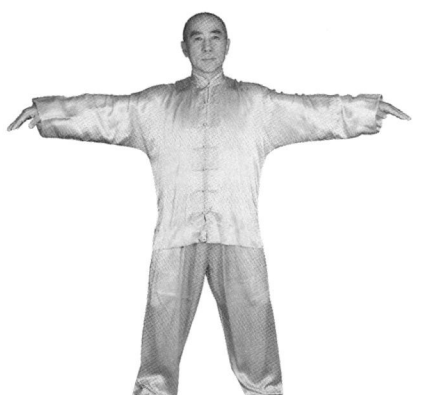

Figure 9-58

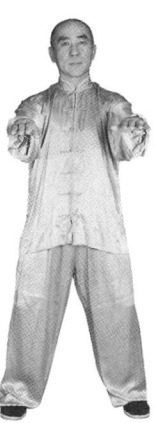

Figure 9-59

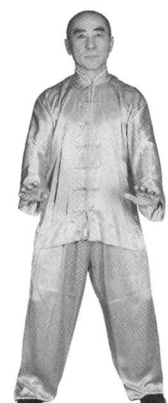

Figure 9-60

Core Form (Figures 9-60 to 9-68)

Right Side (Figures 9-60 to 9-64)

From the position in figure 9-60, as you shift the body center toward the left leg and turn the torso 45 degrees to the left, forming a small bow stance, float both arms up to shoulder height (figure 9-61).

As you turn the torso 45 degrees to the right and shift the body center toward the right leg, swing both arms 45 degrees to the right. While the

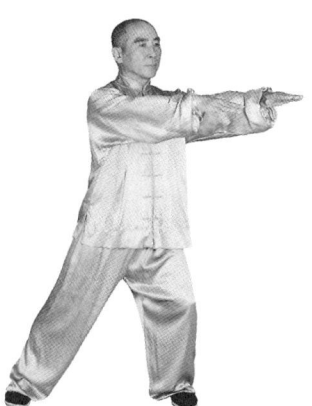

Figure 9-61

right hand continues to circle down to the side of the right hip, palm facing up, bend the left arm, crossing it in front of the chest, palm facing down, and look straight ahead (figure 9-62).

Turn the body so it faces front, and center it by standing with legs shoulder-width apart and knees slightly bent. Simultaneously, the right palm shoots upward to the front center of the face, open palm facing the face, while the inside of the left arm pushes the left hand downward to the level of the abdomen, the left palm facing down (figure 9-63).

When the right palm arrives at forehead level and the left palm arrives at the level of the abdomen, open both elbows and swing the right hand above and in front of the right side of your head with the palm facing up while the left palm moves down and out to the front-left side of the body, palm facing downward (figure 9-64).

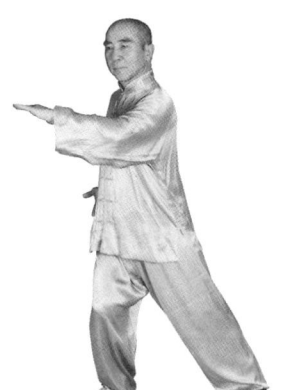
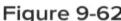
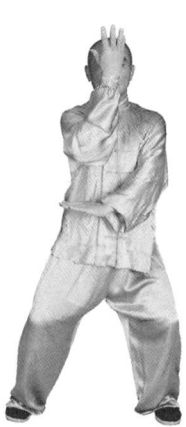
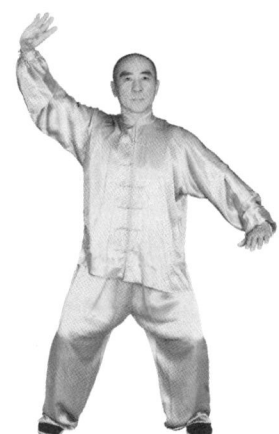

Figure 9-62   Figure 9-63   Figure 9-64

Left Side (Figures 9-64 to 9-68)

As you shift the body center toward the right leg and turn the torso 45 degrees to the right, drop the right hand to the front-right side of the body and float the left hand slightly up to be parallel with the right hand at shoulder height, both palms facing down (figure 9-65).

As you turn the torso 45 degrees to the left and shift the body center toward the slightly bent left leg, forming a left bow stance, swing both arms 45 degrees to the left. Without stopping, let the left hand continue to circle down to the left side of the hip, palm facing up. Bend the right elbow, crossing it in front of the chest with palm facing down, and look straight ahead (figure 9-66).

Turn the body 45 degrees back to center, facing front, knees slightly bent, while the left palm shoots upward, the palm open to the face, and the right hand moves downward to the level of the abdomen, the palm facing down (figure 9-67).

When the left palm is at forehead level and the right palm is at the level of the abdomen, open both elbows outward to have the left hand over the left-front side of the head, palm facing up, while the right hand is out to the front-right side of the body, palm facing downward (figure 9-68).

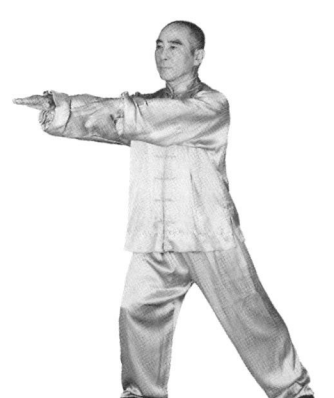 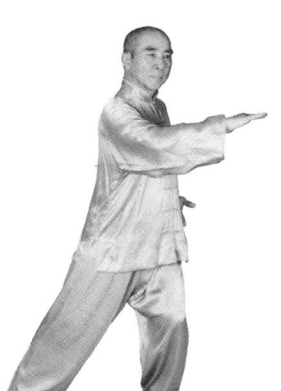 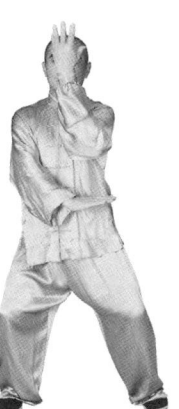 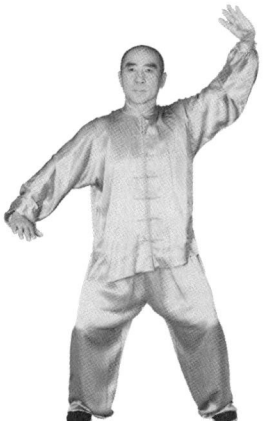

| Figure 9-65 | Figure 9-66 | Figure 9-67 | Figure 9-68 |

Closing Form (Figures 9-68 to 9-74)

From the position in figure 9-68, drop the left hand down to slightly below the shoulder and float the right hand up to the same position, arms out to the sides and both palms facing down (figure 9-69).

Bring the arms to the front in a circular motion, both hands shoulder-width apart and slightly below shoulder height (figure 9-70).

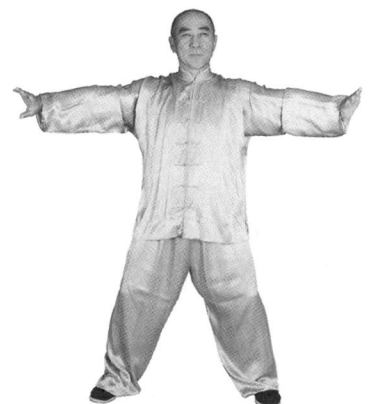 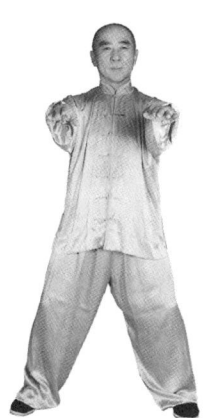

Figure 9-69   Figure 9-70

Gently drop the arms to the sides of the hips, palms facing the hips (figure 9-71).

Circle your arms to shoulder height with palms facing up. Shifting the body center to the right leg, bring the left foot next to the right foot and then center the body evenly (figure 9-72).

Bring both palms to the front of the hips with a curved motion. Turn the palms to face down, then gently push both hands down and let them rest at the sides of the body (figures 9-73 to 9-74).

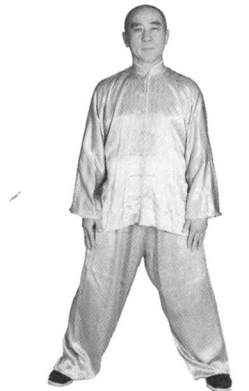
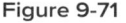

Figure 9-71

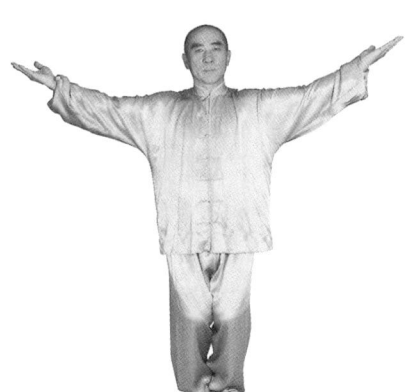

Figure 9-72

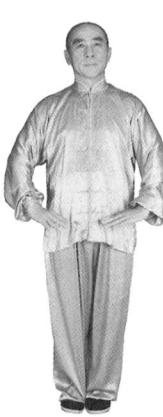

Figure 9-73

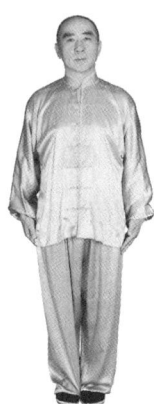

Figure 9-74

⦚ Movement 5: Flying Arrow Chases the Tiger, or Cover Hand and Thrust Fist (Figures 9-74 to 9-94)

Preparatory Posture (Figure 9-74)

While standing, keep your knees slightly bent and sink the body downward, keeping the head, neck, and body upright and holding the head straight up as if suspended from above by a thread. Release all tension from the shoulders and arms, letting the arms hang gently at your sides. Mentally connect all relaxed body parts to your body center (spine and legs), making them a calmly engaged body system. Eyes look straight forward, their gaze like two swords that look through everything before you.

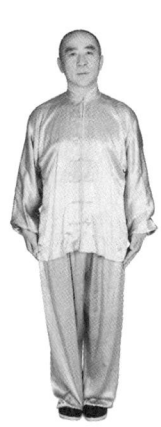

Figure 9-74

Commencing Form (Figures 9-75 to 9-78)

Slowly shift the body center toward the right leg and step to the left, keeping the feet parallel and shoulder-width apart and opening both toes slightly outward (figure 9-75).

Slowly raise the arms to shoulder height, palms facing down, and relax the wrists (figure 9-76).

Without stopping, bring the arms to the front, shoulder-width apart and shoulder height, with the elbows down and the palms relaxed and facing down (figure 9-77).

While bending your legs slowly into a comfortable position, bend and drop the elbows and draw the arms slightly inward, pushing your forearms down to the front of the abdomen. Keep both hands shoulder-width apart (figure 9-78).

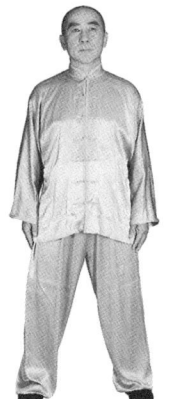

Figure 9-75

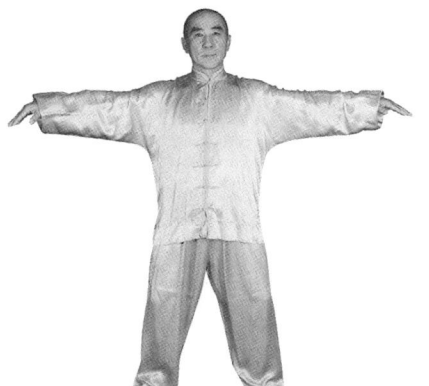

Figure 9-76

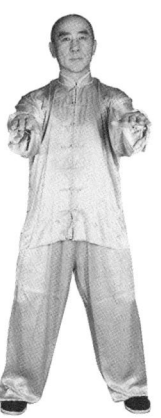

Figure 9-77

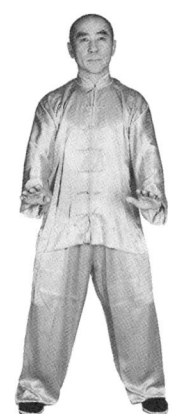

Figure 9-78

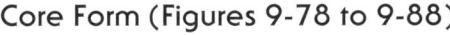

Core Form (Figures 9-78 to 9-88)

Left Side (Figures 9-78 to 9-84)

From the position in figure 9-78, shift the body center to the right leg and turn the body 45 degrees to the right. Push both palms down and slightly back (figure 9-79).

As you shift the body center to between the legs and turn the body to

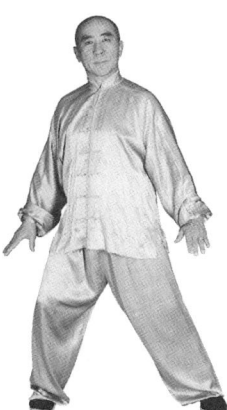

Figure 9-79

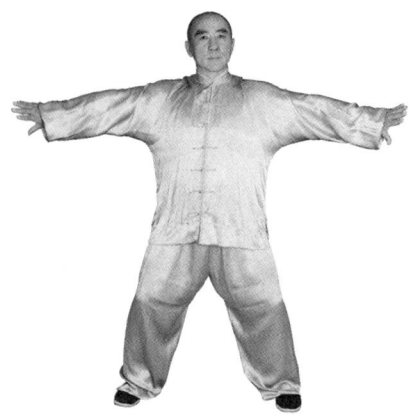

Figure 9-80

face the front, float both arms up to slightly below shoulder height. The arms and body form a slight curve (figure 9-80).

Without stopping, move your arms up in an outward circular movement and bring them together in front in a "V" shape slightly above the shoulders, bending the elbows with palms facing up (figure 9-81).

While turning the torso 45 degrees to the left, shift the body center toward the left leg to form a left bow stance. Simultaneously form a loose fist with the left hand and turn the fist up and draw it back, the side of your fist gently pressed on the navel. At the same time, move the right arm slightly inward to the front of the abdomen, creating a gentle blocking energy, palm facing up and at nose height (figure 9-82).

As you quickly but gently turn the torso 45 degrees to the right, shift the body center toward the right leg to make a right bow stance. Pull the right palm back and make a loose fist to replace the left fist's position at the abdomen, simultaneously rolling the left fist over and throwing it softly out, through turning the body, over the right forearm to nose height (figure 9-83).

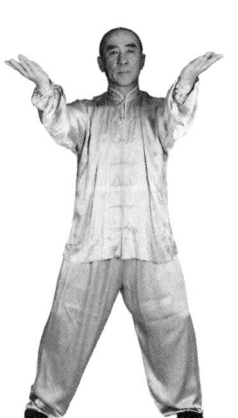

Figure 9-81

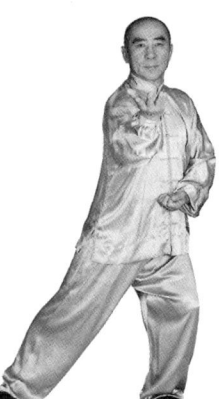

Figure 9-82

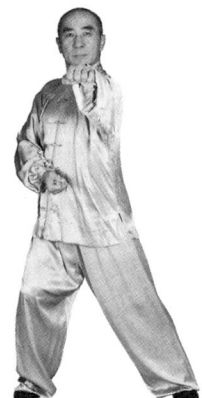

Figure 9-83

Right Side (Figures 9-83 to Figure 9-88)

From the position in figure 9-83, as you shift the body center to the left leg and turn the body 45 degrees to the left, open the fists and push both palms down and slightly back (figure 9-84).

As you shift the body center to between the legs and turn the body to face front, float both arms up to slightly below shoulder height, the arms and body forming a slight curve (figure 9-85).

Without stopping, move your arms up in an outward circular movement and bring them together in front of you into a "V" shape slightly above the shoulder, bending the elbows, and the palms facing up (figure 9-86).

While turning the torso 45 degrees to the right, shift the body center toward the right leg, making a right bow stance. Simultaneously form a loose fist with the right hand, palm side facing up. Draw the fist back, the end of your fist gently pressed on the navel. At the same time, move the left arm slightly inward to the front of the abdomen to create a gentle blocking energy, the palm facing up and at nose height (figure 9-87).

As you shift the body center to the left leg to make a left bow stance, quickly but gently turn the torso 45 degrees to the left. Pull the left palm back and change it to a loose fist to replace the right fist's position, simultaneously rolling the right fist over and throwing it out softly, through turning the body, over the left forearm to nose height (figure 9-88).

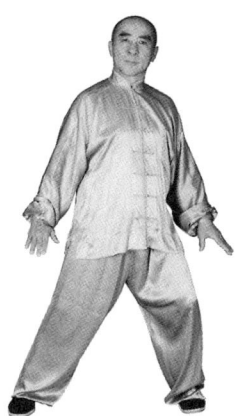

Figure 9-84

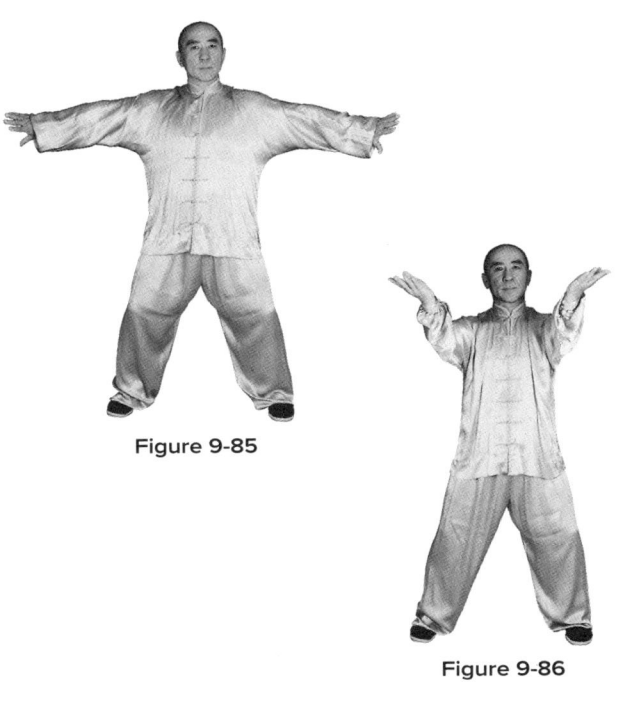

Figure 9-85

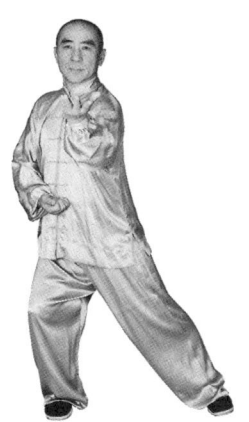

Figure 9-86

Figure 9-87

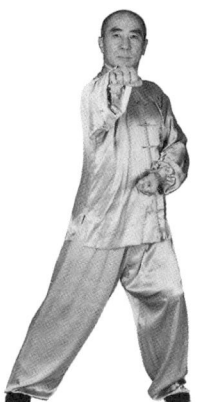

Figure 9-88

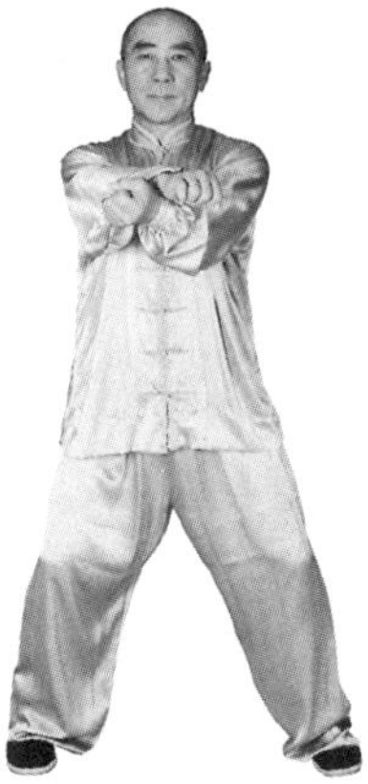

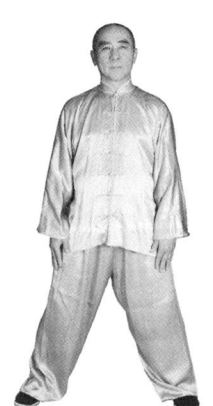

Figure 9-89

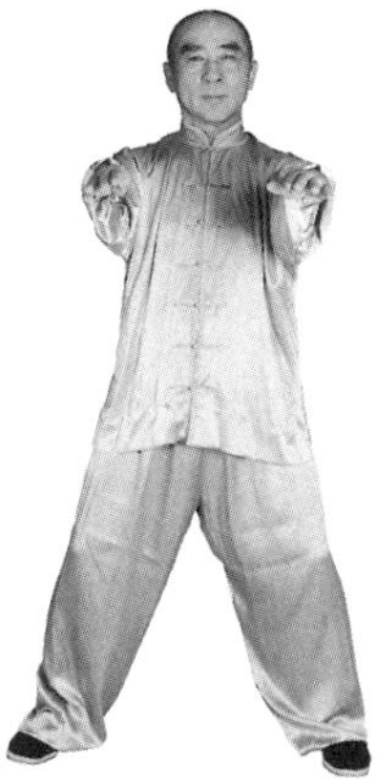

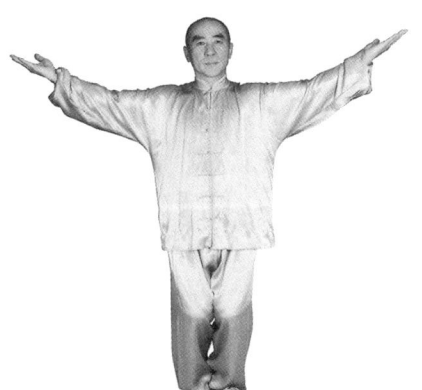

Figure 9-90

Closing Form (Figures 9-88 to 9-94)

From the position in figure 9-88, rotate the body to face the front and reach the left fist out under the right, the left fist facing up (figure 9-89).

Open both arms to shoulder width and rotate the palms to face down, thumbs inward (figure 9-90).

Gently drop the arms to the sides of the hips, palms facing the hips (figure 9-91).

Circle your arms to shoulder height, palms facing up. While shifting the body center to the right leg, step the left foot next to the right foot (figure 9-92).

Bring both palms to the front of the chest in a curved motion. Turn the palms to face down and gently push both hands down the front of the body to the level of the hips, bringing them to rest at the sides of the body (figures 9-93 to 9-94).

Figure 9-91

Figure 9-92

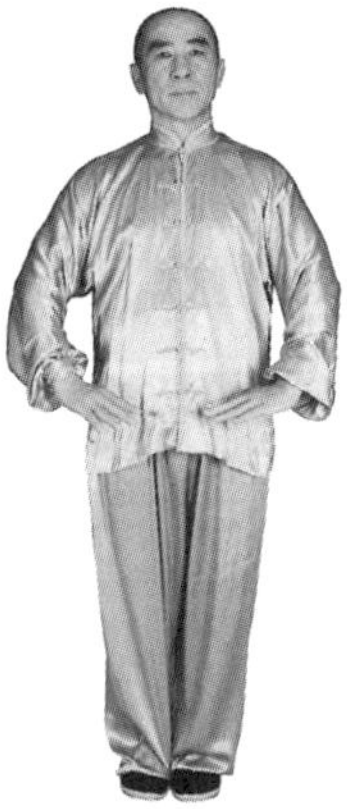

Figure 9-93

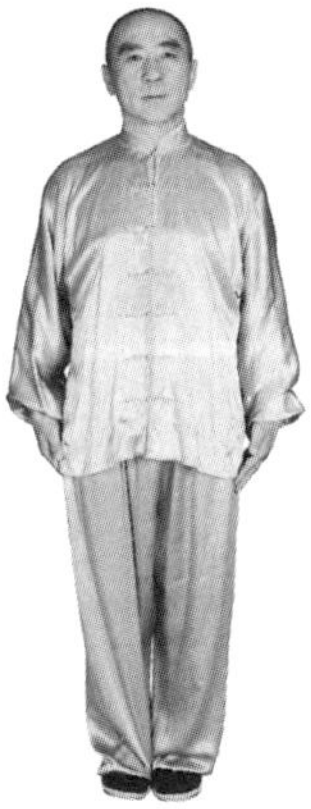

Figure 9-94

⦂ Movement 6: Needle at the Bottom of the Ocean (Figures 9-94 to 9-115)

Preparatory Posture (Figure 9-94)

While standing, keep your knees slightly bent and sink the body downward. Keep the head, neck, and body upright and hold the head straight up as if suspended from above by a thread. Release all tension from the shoulders and arms, letting the arms hang gently at your sides. Mentally connect all relaxed body parts to your body center (spine and legs), making them a calmly engaged body system. Eyes look straightforward, their gaze like two swords that look through everything before you.

Commencing Form (Figures 9-95 to 9-98)

Slowly shift the body center toward the right leg and step to the left, keeping the feet parallel and shoulder-width apart and opening both toes slightly outward (figure 9-95).

Slowly raise both arms to shoulder height, palms facing down, and relax the wrists (figure 9-96).

Without stopping, bring the arms to the front, shoulder-width apart and shoulder height, the elbows down and the palms relaxed and facing down (figure 9-97).

While slightly bending your legs into a comfortable position, bend and drop the elbows and draw the arms slightly inward, pushing your forearms down to the front of the abdomen. Keep both hands shoulder-width apart (figure 9-98).

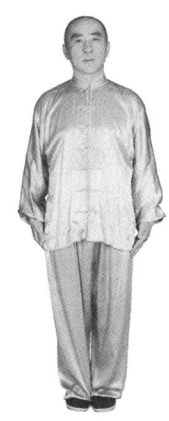

Figure 9-94

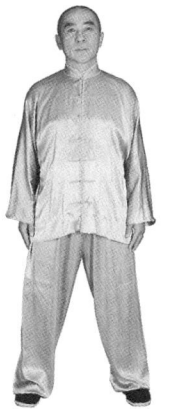

Figure 9-95

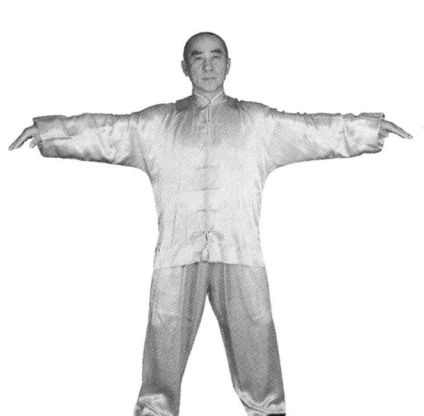

Figure 9-96

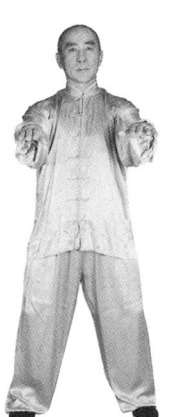

Figure 9-97

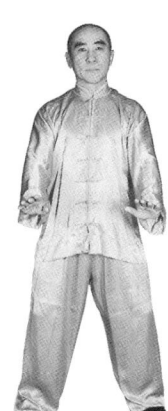

Figure 9-98

Core Form (Figures 9-98 to 9-109)

The Right Side (Figures 9-98 to 9-103)

From figure 9-98, as you rotate the torso slightly to the right, slide your right hand down with the palm facing up and to the side; at the same time, the left arm floats up to the left side of the forehead (figure 9-99).

As you swing the right hand in an outward and upward curve to the front of your right shoulder with the palm facing up, the left hand continues the blocking motion downward to the front of the navel, the palm turned to face up (figure 9-100).

As the torso turns 45 degrees to the left and the center shifts to the left leg to form a left bow stance, pull the left hand across the abdomen and swing it out and up to the left side of the body, the palm facing up, while the right hand blocks across the face to the left (figure 9-101).

The left hand continues to float up at the side of the body to pass the shoulder and arrive at the side of the head, thumb pointing up and palm facing the left temple. At the same time, the right hand circles down to the left side of the hip with fingers slightly pointing down (figure 9-102).

While turning the torso 45 degrees to the right and shifting the body center to the right leg to a make right bow stance, move the right hand across the body to the right side of the hip, the palm facing down, and strike down the left hand to the left, the thumb pointing up and the fingers pointing 45 degrees downward (figure 9-103).

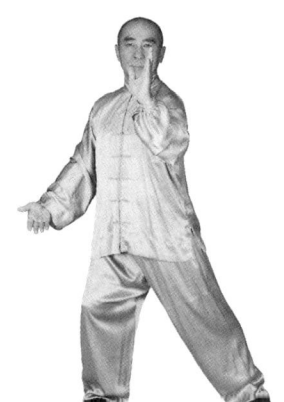

Figure 9-99

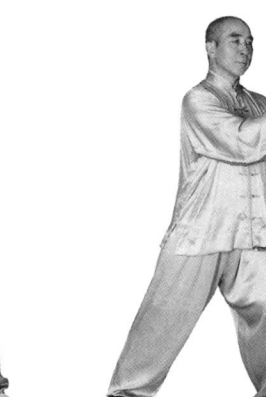

Figure 9-100

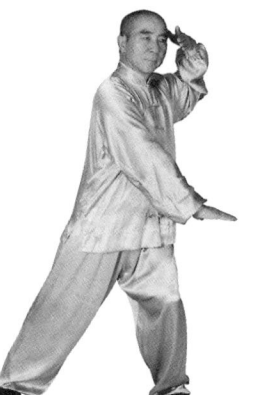

Figure 9-101

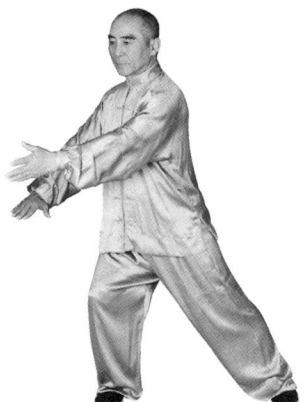

Figure 9-102

Figure 9-103

The Left Side (Figures 9-103 to 9-109)

From the position in figure 9-103, pull the left hand across the abdomen and swing the right hand out and up, the palm facing up (figure 9-104).

As the torso turns 45 degrees to the left, shift the body center to the left leg while the right hand floats up and moves across the face to the left (figure 9-105).

As the left hand continues to pull to the left and floats up at the side of the body, the right hand moves down to the front of the navel, the palm face up (figure 9-106).

As the torso turns 45 degrees to the right, shift the body center to the right leg. Pull the right hand across the abdomen and swing it out and upward to the right side of the body, the palm facing up, while the left palm moves across the face to the right (figure 9-107).

The right hand floats up the side of the body to the side of the head, thumb pointing up and palm facing the right temple; at the same time, the left hand circles down to the right side of the hip with fingers slightly pointing down (figure 9-108).

While turning the torso 45 degrees to the left and shifting the body center to the left to make a right bow stance, move the left hand across the body to the right side of the hip with the palm facing down and strike the right hand down to the right, the thumb pointing up and fingers pointing 45 degrees downward (figure 9-109).

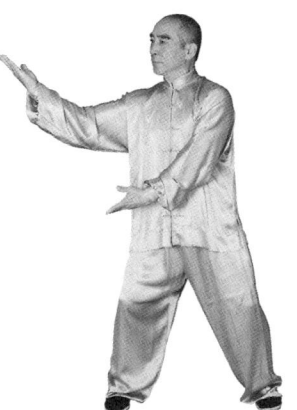

Figure 9-104

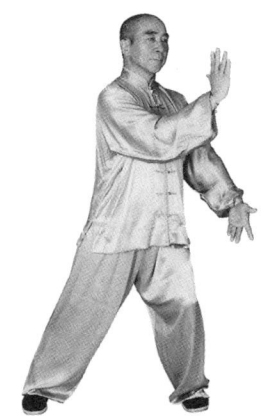

Figure 9-105

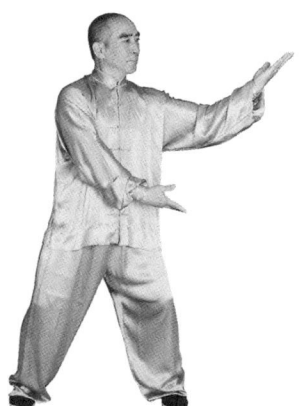

Figure 9-106

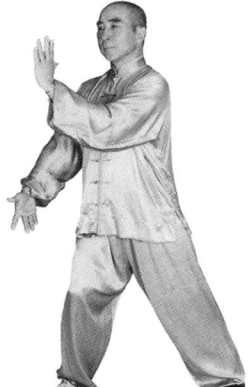

Figure 9-107

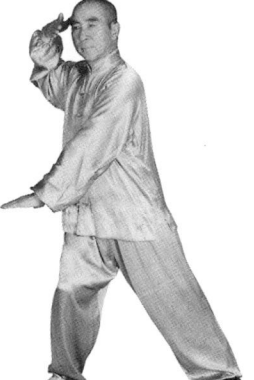

Figure 9-108

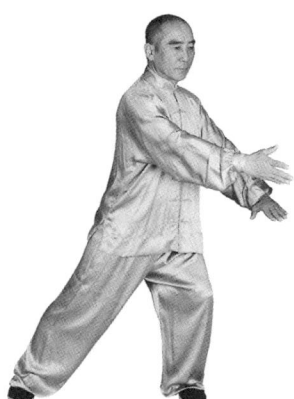

Figure 9-109

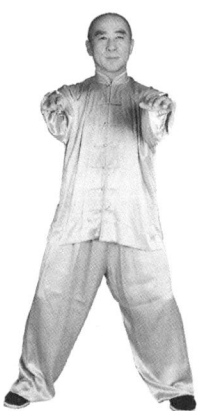

Figure 9-110

Closing Form (Figures 9-109 to 9-115)

From the position in figure 9-109, rotate the body to face the front and swing the left hand to the left side; extend both arms at shoulder level, palms facing down (figure 110).

Bring the arms to the front in a circular motion; both hands are shoulder-width apart and slightly below shoulder height (figure 9-111).

Gently drop the arms to the sides of the hips, the palms facing the hips (figure 9-112).

Circle your arms to shoulder height with palms facing up. While shifting the body center to the right leg, step the left foot next to the right foot (figure 9-113).

Bring both palms to the front of the chest in a curved motion, turning the palms face down, and gently push both hands down from the front of the body to rest at the sides (figures 9-114 to 9-115).

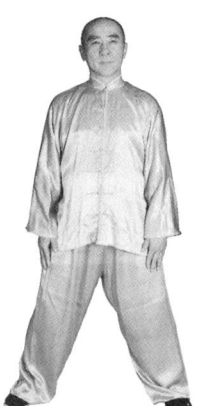

Figure 9-111

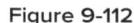

Figure 9-112

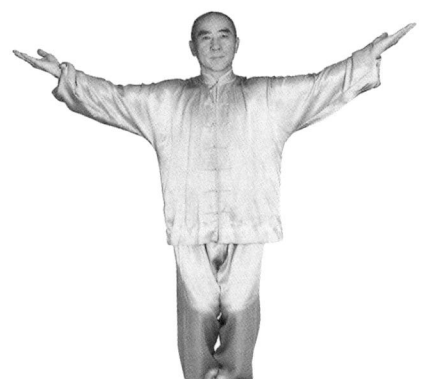

Figure 9-113

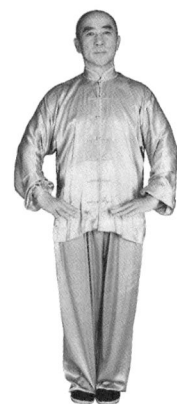

Figure 9-114

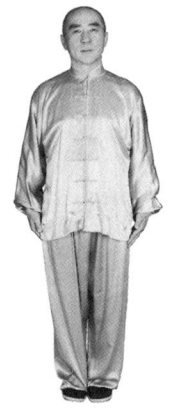

Figure 9-115

: Movement 7: Bend the Bow to the Catch Tiger (Figures 9-115 to 9-134)

Preparatory Posture (Figure 9-115)

While standing, keep your knees slightly bent and sink the body downward. Keep the head, neck, and body upright and hold the head straight up as if suspended from above by a thread. Release all tension from the shoulders and arms, letting the arms hang gently at your sides. Mentally connect all relaxed body parts to your body center (spinal cord and two legs), making them a calmly engaged body system. Eyes look straight forward, their gaze like two swords that look through everything before you.

Commencing Form (Figures 9-116 to 9-119)

Slowly shift the body center toward the right leg, step to the left, and keep the feet parallel and shoulder-width apart, opening both toes slightly outward (figure 9-116).

Slowly raise both arms to the shoulder height, palms facing down, and relax the wrists (figure 9-117).

Without stopping, bring the arms to the front, shoulder-width apart and shoulder height, with the elbows down and palms relaxed and facing down (figure 9-118).

While bending your legs slowly into a comfortable position, bend and drop the elbows and draw the arms slightly inward, pushing your forearms down to the front of the abdomen and keeping both hands shoulder-width apart (figure 9-119).

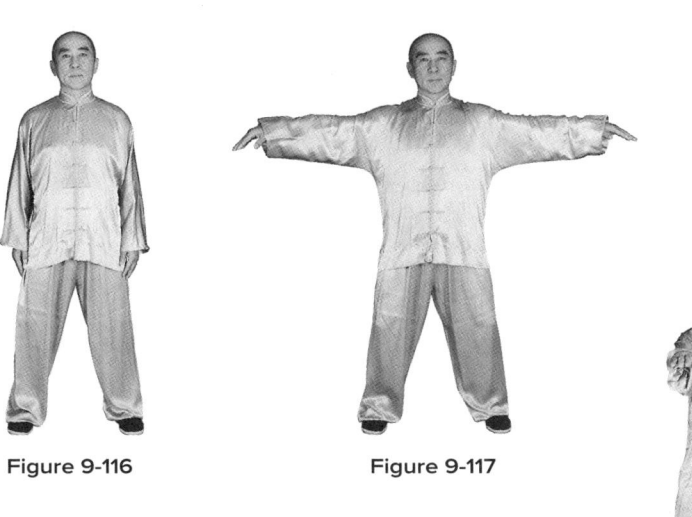

Figure 9-116   Figure 9-117

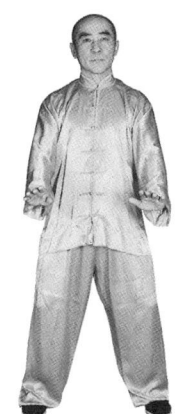

Figure 9-118   Figure 9-119

Core Form (Figures 9-119 to 9-128)

The Right Side (Figures 9-119 to 9-123)

From the position in figure 9-119, as you shift the body center to the left leg and turn the torso 45 degrees to the left, bend your elbows slightly and, following the energy of the body's rotation, float the arms up 45 degrees to the left, the fingers pointing straight. Both arms are shoulder-width apart and at shoulder height, palms facing down, the elbows pointing slightly downward (figure 9-120).

As you rotate your torso 45 degrees to the right and shift the body center to the right, making a right bow stance, follow the energy of the body's rotation and slowly swing both arms down across the diaphragm, palms facing down and to the right side of the body (figure 9-121).

Without stopping, both arms float upward in a circle to the right side of the head; at the same time, make loose fists with both hands, bend both elbows, and place the left fist in front of the right elbow, with the heart of the right fist facing up slightly and the heart of the left fist facing right (figure 9-122).

While maintaining a right bow stance, turn the body slightly to the left, simultaneously striking out both fists 45 degrees to the left, the right fist slightly above the right forehead and the left fist away from the body at nose height, left elbow bent (figure 9-123).

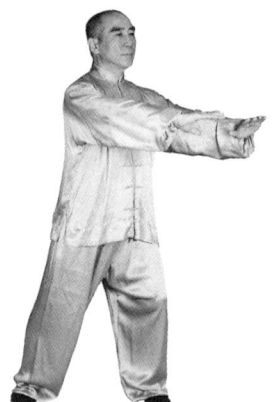

Figure 9-120

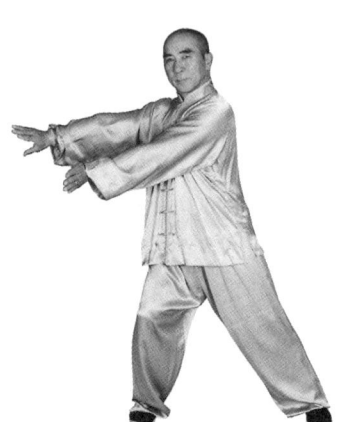

Figure 9-121

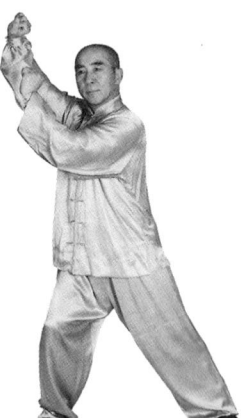

Figure 9-122

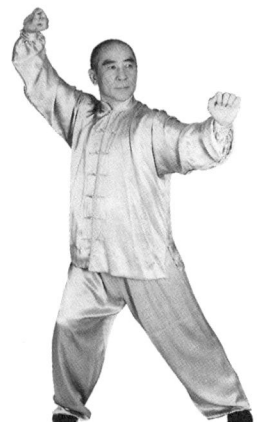

Figure 9-123

The Left Side (Figures 9-123 to 9-128)

Shift the body center to between the legs, turn the body to face front, and extend both hands to the sides at shoulder height. Arms and body form a curve (figure 9-124).

As you rotate the body center to the right leg and face 45 degrees to the right, swing the left arm to the right, parallel with the right arm. Both arms are shoulder-width apart and at shoulder height, elbows slightly bent and palms facing down (figure 9-125).

As you rotate your torso 45 degrees to the left and shift the body center to the left leg, making a left bow stance, follow the energy of the body's rotation and slowly swing both arms down across the diaphragm, palms facing down and at the right side of the body (figure 9-126).

Without stopping, both arms float upward in a circle to the left side of the head; at the same time, make the palms into loose fists, bend both elbows, and place the right fist in front of the left elbow, with the heart of the left fist slightly facing up and the heart of the right fist facing left (figure 9-127).

While maintaining a left bow stance, turn the body slightly to the right, simultaneously striking both fists out 45 degrees to the right, the left fist slightly above the left forehead and the right fist away from the body at nose height with the elbow bent (figure 9-128).

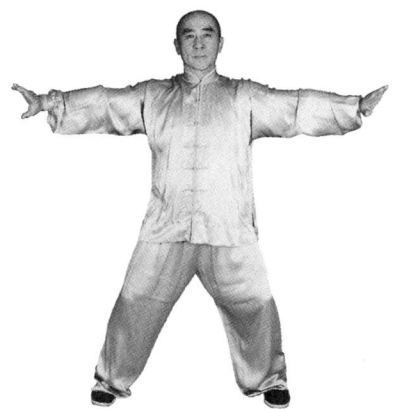

Figure 9-124

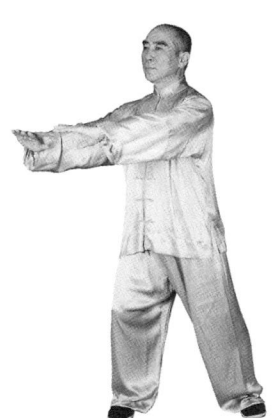

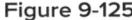

Figure 9-125

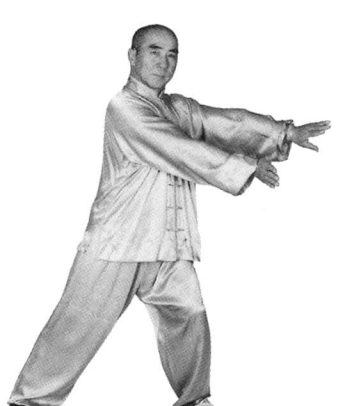

Figure 9-126

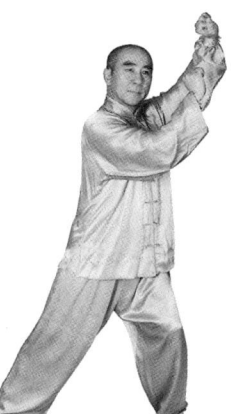

Figure 9-127

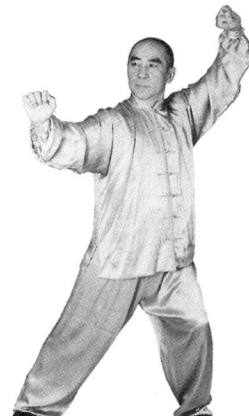

Figure 9-128

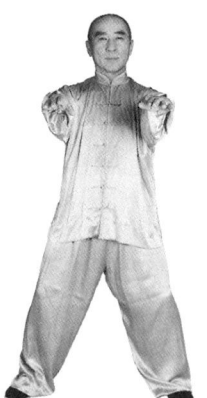

Figure 9-129

Closing Form (Figures 9-128 to 9-134)

From the position in figure 9-128, rotate the body to face the front and swing the left hand to the left; extend the arms at shoulder level, palms facing down (figure 9-129).

Bring the arms to the front in a circular motion; both hands are shoulder-width apart and slightly below shoulder height (figure 9-130).

Gently drop the arms to the sides of the hips, the palms facing the hips (figure 9-131).

Circle your arms to shoulder height with palms facing up. While shifting the body center to the right leg, step the left foot next to the right, slightly bending the knees (figure 9-132).

Bring both palms to the front of the chest in a curved motion, turning the palms face down, and gently push both hands down from the front of the body to rest at the sides (figures 9-133 to 9-134).

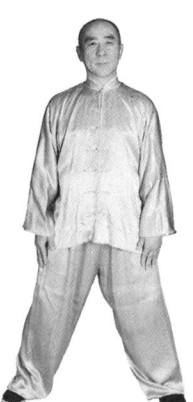

Figure 9-130

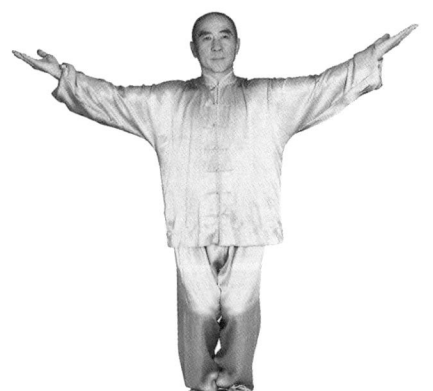

Figure 9-131

Figure 9-132

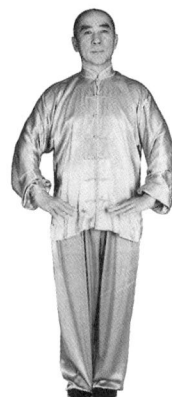

Figure 9-133

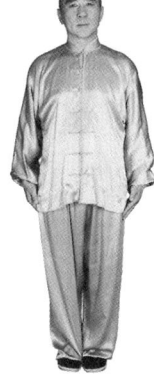

Figure 9-134

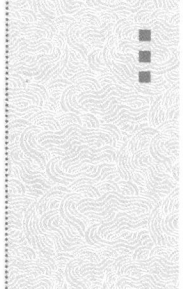

ABOUT THE COMMENCING AND CLOSING FORMS

See the last section of chapter 5, "The Commencing and Closing Forms," to learn more about the symbolism and function of the opening and closing forms.

10

Conclusion

The Essence of Flow

THE MIND is at the core of our transformation through Tai Chi Chuan. To empower the body, one must empower the mind. A calm and flowing mind can unify body parts so that they work harmoniously within a gently flowing system.

Tai Chi Chuan's inclusivity inspired the development of wheelchair adaptive Tai Chi Chuan programs for people of all physical conditions. The positive reception of these programs worldwide is particularly encouraging in a social context in which ableism and ageism have intensified the challenges of the differently abled.

The stories in this book are not about disability or ability. They are reminders of the power of our mind and how each of the Tai Chi Chuan practice modalities can effectively transform our resources into great achievements, regardless of our physical conditions and abilities. Participants have kindly shared with us the many ways in which adaptive Tai Chi Chuan practices empower them, meet their needs, and support their values by giving them a sense of camaraderie and unity, renewed spirit, healing, ability, power, connection to nature, beauty, and peace.

A SENSE OF HEALING

The positive impact of practice on the mind and body is one of the most popular benefits shared by participants. They report reduced physical pain, an increased range of motion, and improvement in their general well-being, sleep, and mental focus. A practitioner said that doing wheelchair Tai Chi was one of the few occasions when he did not feel his body pain. Some participants who did not use a wheelchair but enrolled in the class due to their back and leg-joint injuries told us that the practice helped ease their fear of body movement (kinesiophobia) and helped them regain their confidence in moving. One participant added, "The practice brought me back to my golf game."

Ms. Z. is a female veteran who endures both physical and mental challenges. After a few years of participation, she reported,

> I have several problems, ranging from back problems, some paresthesia, and depression, and this exacerbates my PTSD. So when I come here, it's like a reprieve from everything else. It helps ground and center me. I often feel numb to the world, what's going on, and just being here helps me reconnect with myself because you have no choice but to feel what you're doing while you're doing it. It's very thought-provoking and body-inducing. My first time here, I came in a wheelchair, and now I'm using a cane. It's been amazing.

Mr. K is a veteran of the Korean and Vietnam wars. He told the group,

> I was doing the practices in a wheelchair. Now I am up and doing it. When I make my turns, I have to take baby steps for my balance, but because of the camaraderie of everyone I see, I am not doing it in a wheelchair. I use a walker. This program gives me two things every day: I can see another sunset and I can see another sunrise.

A SENSE OF ABILITY

A sense of ability is fundamental to our motivation and well-being and shapes how we experience and engage with the world. When we believe we are capable, we're more likely to take on challenges, pursue goals, and actively engage with life. The positive changes in mental and physical well-being experienced by many participants contributed to their enthusiasm and motivation. For many participants, turning in wheelchair Tai Chi Chuan movements gives them a sense of ability and power.

An older veteran shared, "When I started I could hardly get out of my chair and had to have people around me; now I can stand up and even walk some. Doing all the moves helps me focus on my thought processes." Another wheelchair Tai Chi practitioner from Tianjin, China, told us, "Being able to do Tai Chi was the only thing I dreamed I could do, and I am doing it. Everyone around me is so proud of me and has begun to see me differently."

A SENSE OF RENEWED WARRIOR SPIRIT

Many participants with disabilities, and healthcare providers, said that low self-esteem is quite common among individuals with severe physical disabilities. Losing one's sense of value because of disability and enduring pain kept many people less socially engaged. The gentle, circular, and flowing movements of adaptive Tai Chi can provide participants with a feeling of renewed body and spirit. One veteran said that sitting in a chair, flowing with gentle martial-arts movements alongside others, "is the only time I do not feel disabled." The enduring appeal of martial arts stems from its ability to physically, culturally, and philosophically support our innate drive to overcome challenges on various levels. Another veteran said, "The slow, gentle, and circular movements help me embrace and redirect forces, which is also the beauty of martial-arts application in life."

A SENSE OF CAMARADERIE AND UNITY

One of the unique features of inclusive Tai Chi Chuan is that the seven sequenced movements can be practiced in standing, sitting, walking, or wheelchair modalities. In group practice, participants can choose any of the four modalities and synchronize each movement while moving together in unison. One veteran told me during a practice break that when she saw everyone in class—in a wheelchair or standing or sitting, using one arm or two arms—flowing together in sync with the music, she felt so happy and empowered that she forgot where she was and why she was there.

Many veteran participants reported that the camaraderie developed during practice made them want to return after each class. There were no differences in physical and health conditions and no social distinctions when they practiced together. They shared the collective flow, a unified energy that felt beautiful and powerful.

A Vietnam vet, Mr. M, said during a class discussion,

> The class was very enjoyable. Not only did Tai Chi exercises help me physically and mentally, but I found it almost as rewarding to meet and connect with other veterans. The brotherhood that we have as veterans. It's special and like nothing else I've done in life.

Another veteran commented, "Doing Tai Chi with others makes me smile, helps me feel calm, and gives me a sense of peace."

A SENSE OF CONNECTION TO NATURE

As George Lakoff, the author of *Metaphors We Live By*, puts it: "Our ordinary conceptual system, in terms of which we both think and act, is fundamentally metaphorical. . . . Metaphor is thus imaginative rationality." Metaphors shape our perceptions about life and the world around us. Positive metaphors that convey uplifting, inspiring, or optimistic ideas and images can evoke feelings of hope, growth, and healing, and can communicate complex ideas and concerns in a more engaging and relatable manner. Over the years, many healthcare providers have shared their positive experiences using metaphors in their clinical practice.

A psychologist at a VA medical center in Florida shared, "When emphasizing the natural, as in "sit like a mountain, stand like a tree, flow like a river," I found many participants were able to increase their sense of internal local control, self-efficacy, and self-empowerment." A physical therapist at a VA medical center in California said, "Picturing nature or observing a movement that simulates a natural activity in nature helps participants to learn postures and create flowing motions. It allows participants to understand the motions and move easily and with less frustration or pain." And an occupational therapist at VA medical center in Colorado said, "These metaphors offer veterans a way to externalize and explore their emotions, making them more tangible and manageable."

A SENSE OF BEAUTY AND POWER

During the instructional training for 140 healthcare providers at ten VA medical centers in 2022, we conducted a small study to explore the people's initial impressions of wheelchair Tai Chi Chuan. Before beginning each of the ten training sessions, we demonstrated the seven-posture inclusive Tai Chi Chuan program using the wheelchair modality. Then we asked the healthcare providers to list three short phrases or words that best describe their impressions of the demonstration. Dr. Danielle Lauber, the program evaluator, did a statistical analysis of the lists and identified five major categories of impressions: flow, power, calm, mindfulness, and aesthetics. Under "aesthetics," there were words such as "artistic," "beautiful," and "graceful."

Conventionally, such impressions are least likely to be associated with wheelchair movements. The prevalent use of social categories such as "disability" or "disabled body" often denotes a negative impression of differently abled people with different physical conditions. The thoughtful design of this adaptive Tai Chi Chuan program makes an assistive device such as a wheelchair a tool for body flow and changes our perception about its function while promoting a positive impression of the practitioner and their participation.

A wheelchair Tai Chi practitioner from Shanghai, China, said this: "When I practice wheelchair Tai Chi, I feel like I'm flying with my chair. I feel so free and powerful."

INVITING FLOW TO THE MIND, BODY, AND SPIRIT

Being in flow is a way of describing Tai Chi Chuan movement. It is also how we describe nature, the way something is beautiful, the way of music, the way of a good story, the way of a good conversation, and when things move forward smoothly. As one veteran participant echoed, "Flowing is not just a principle of the Tai Chi Chuan movement, it is also a way of life."

However, in the natural and social world, flow is the process of cultivating power and the result of power. In the natural world, flow is said to be the way of nature, the Dao prescribed by the ancient thinkers. In the social world, the power of making things flow comes from either collective or individual effort. Flow, power, and calm perfectly characterize conventional Tai Chi Chuan movements and their approach to cultivating power. In reading this book, I hope you've embraced how unique it is that these words can be used to describe adaptive Tai Chi Chuan. This is an inspired flip from conventional thinking in which the wheelchair is associated with disability rather than ability. Adaptive Tai Chi Chuan promotes a sense of transformation, power, and beauty by making chair, body, and breath move in one unified, gentle flow.

In Tai Chi Chuan, flow creates power. In an adaptive modality, short phrases to guide participants through gently circular movements—such as "yielding is to redirect," "without folding there is no unfolding," "crisis is opportunity," and "the end of a circle is the beginning of the next"—make the flow even more intimately meaningful to participants and their efforts to engage with their challenges in a world in which there is often very little flow. Over the years, many participants have told us that they felt these phrases were directed at them personally and that hearing them was empowering. "I felt like I just had a kind of therapy like no other," one commented.

Flow is at the heart of Tai Chi Chuan's enduring legacy. During an interview with Pierre Berton in 1971, Bruce Lee stated his philosophy of flexibility, adaptability, and the power of being fluid in practicing martial arts and engaging in life. "Empty your mind, be formless, shapeless—like water. Now you put water in a cup, and it becomes the cup; you put water into a bottle, and it becomes the bottle; you put it in a teapot, and it becomes the teapot. Now water can flow, or it can crash. Be water, my friend."

To conclude this book in a flowing style, I'd like to offer my invitation: let's flow with Tai Chi Chuan movements together, regardless of our different physical conditions. Be well, my friend!

Acknowledgments

WRITING THIS BOOK would not have been possible without the support, encouragement, collaboration, guidance, and inspiration of so many individuals and organizations. My heartfelt and sincere gratitude goes to the following:

My later teachers Masters Xue-xi Fan, Gong-wei Xu, Gui-xiang Kan, and Shu-ren Wei who taught me the way of martial arts and inspired me to embrace and transform all challenges in life through martial arts and Tai Chi practice.

Xue-dong Wang, Bao-yu, Tian, of the China Administration Center for Paralympics Sports (CACPS) and Professor Yu-yang Zang of Nanjing University for conducting the first National Wheelchair Tai Chi Chuan Instructor Training Workshop in 2006 and organizing the wheelchair Tai Chi demonstration at the 2008 Paralympics.

Feng Chen, Xiao-li Chen, and Cheng-lin Zhang of CACPS for their efforts conducting interviews with wheelchair Tai Chi practitioners across the country. The data they generated was invaluable to understanding how participants experience and perceive wheelchair Tai Chi.

Dr. William Johnson, Dr. Nancy Fell, Dr. Janet Secrest, and Lauren Barlew of the University of Tennessee at Chattanooga (UTC), and Dr. Glenn Haban of Siskin Hospital for Physical Rehabilitation for conducting the first study exploring the benefits of wheelchair Tai Chi practice for people with ambulatory disability due to spinal cord injuries/diseases.

Dr. Katherine Lindgren, Dr. Miriam Zwitter, and Dr. Christine of UTC for inviting me to participate in three federally funded projects, which allowed me to develop the population-based adaptive Tai Chi program and explore its effects on participants.

Dr. Danielle Lauber, Sharon Stephens, Charles Noel, and Terry Mahone of Tennessee Valley Healthcare System, and Dr. William Johnson for working with healthcare providers and veterans to explore the feasibility, applicability, and methods of employing adaptive Tai Chi programs for veterans with ambulatory disability.

The Adaptive Sports Grant Program of the U. S. Department of Veterans Affairs for providing the project seven consecutive years of funding. These funds allowed the project team to conduct 107 training courses of the Inclusive Tai Chi Chuan program for healthcare providers and host adaptive Tai Chi classes for hundreds of veterans with disabilities across the nation.

The Adaptive Tai Chi International instructors who assisted with the instructional training and conducted hundreds of hours of in-person and virtual training for healthcare providers and veterans nationwide: Tag George, Robin George, Beth Herring, Jami Lowery, Chang Phuong, David Prestridge, Joshua Schklar, Gregory H. Schmidt, and Karen Wilson.

Colleagues at UTC who contributed to the project behind the scenes, including Michaella Ace, Mckenzie Gregg, Dr. Liz Hathaway, Hannah Jeffery, Katelyn Myers, Pat Ormond, Jacob Peterson, Dr. Darrell Walsh, and many others. Their findings from conducting surveys, interviews, and data analysis not only helped improve the program but also enriched this book.

All who shared their stories of making life meaningful, graceful, engaged, and harmonious despite facing the many extraordinary challenges of disability. Their stories orientated the approach of this inclusive Tai Chi program and also inspired me to write this book.

Dr. William Johnson, Steve Long, and Suzanne Long, for their collaboration and support in developing and implementing the Inclusive Tai Chi training program for vulnerable populations.

UTC and my colleagues whose support was instrumental in helping me complete this book. I am immensely grateful to the university grant specialists Todd Moore-doman and Ashely Ledford.

My colleagues Dr. Pam Ashmore and Dr. Lynn Purkey, Dr. Melissa Jarrell, and Dr. Pam Riggs-Gelasco whose care and support made it all possible.

Paul Mcgurik and Megan Lane, two great friends whose encouragement, knowledge, and creative thinking were instrumental in helping me overcome writer's block. I truly appreciate the time they spent listening and brainstorming with me whenever I needed.

My editor, Rochelle Bourgault, whose keen insights and meticulous attention to detail helped shape this manuscript into its final form. Her guidance has been invaluable.

The incredibly talented photographers Ann Jackson and Rainn Jackson for their exceptional photos that brought this book to life.

Beth Frankl, executive editor of Shambhala Publications, and members of the editorial team for helping bring this book to fruition. Their knowledge on the subject matter, thoughtfulness, dedication, creativity, and caring guidance made the revision process a breeze.

My family who are owed my largest debt. They not only tolerated my frequent absences from my busy training and travel schedule but also provided their unwavering support and encouragement throughout the journey. Their patient understanding was my anchor during long nights of writing and revision.

Finally, my readers. I hope you will find this book helpful in your effort to transform challenges into strength, the Tai Chi way!

Appendix: Full Sequences

Wheelchair Tai Chi Chuan

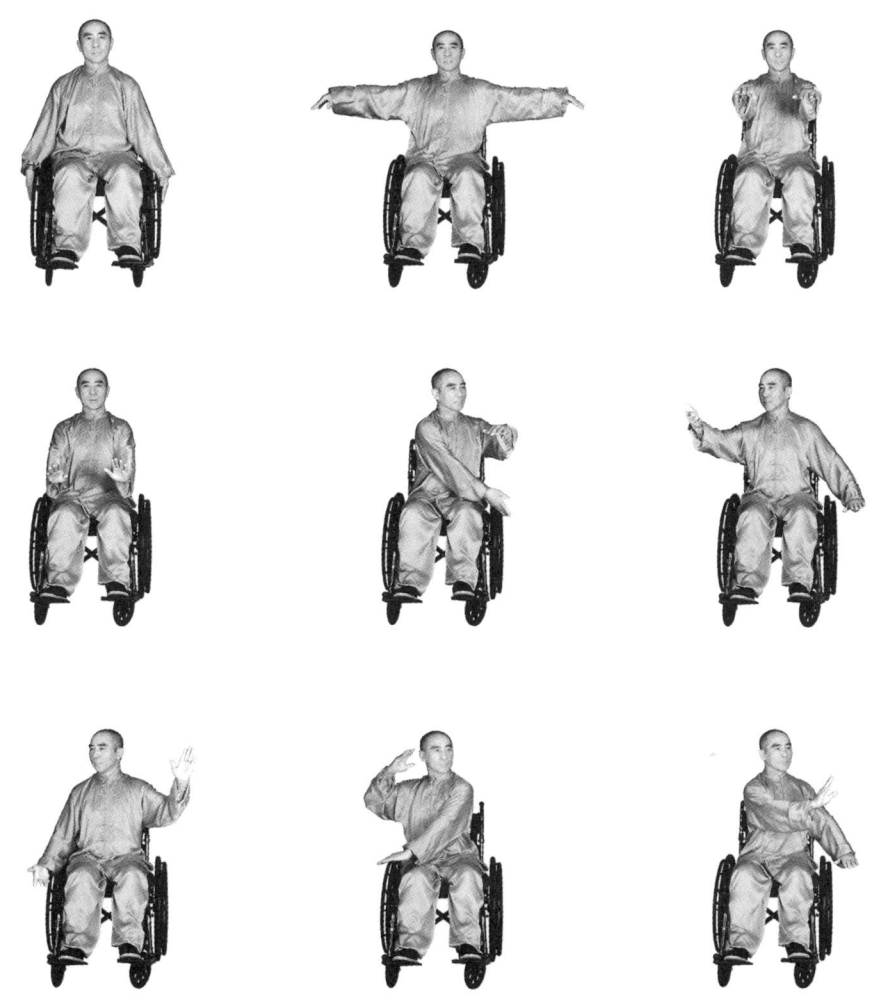

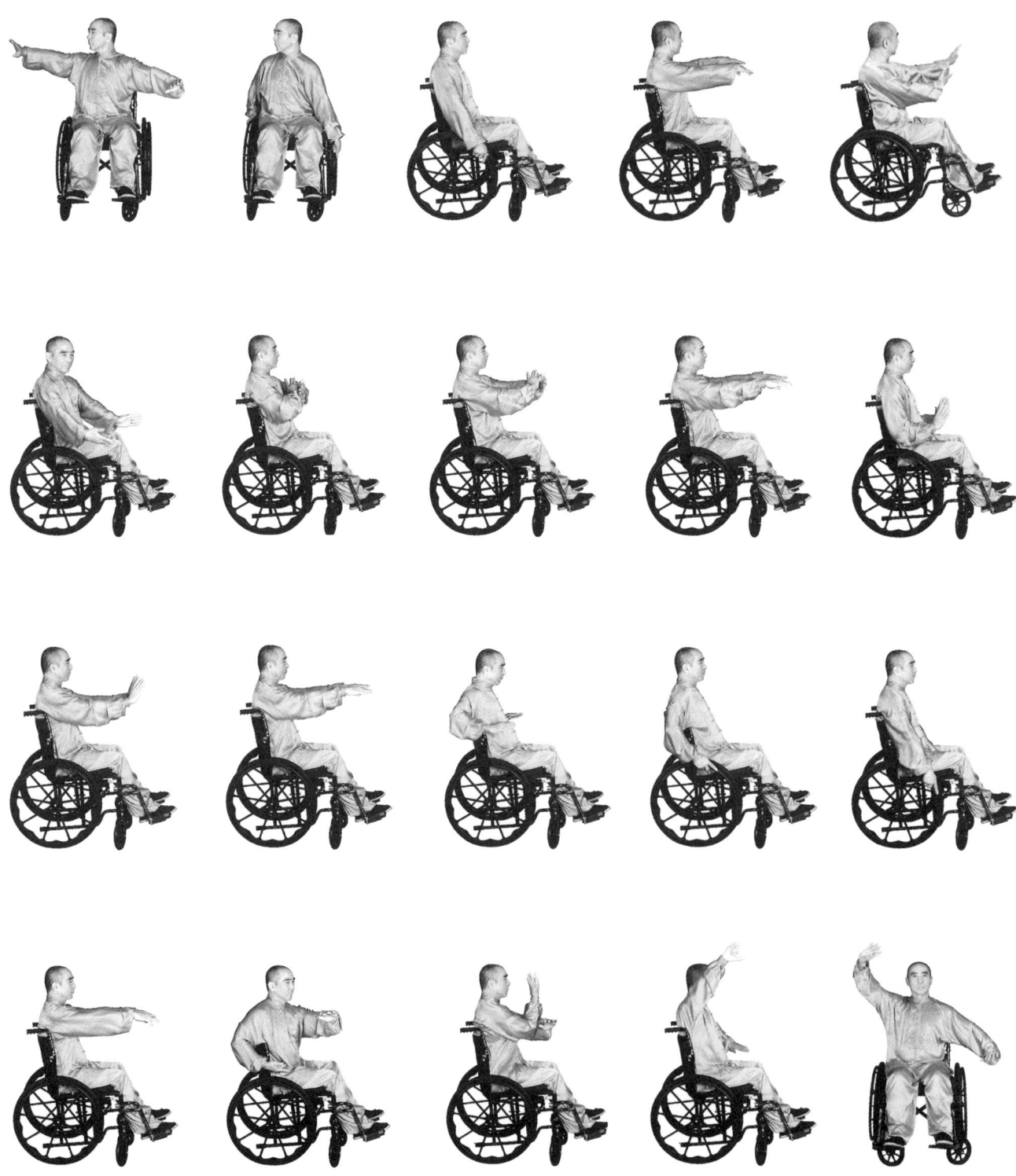

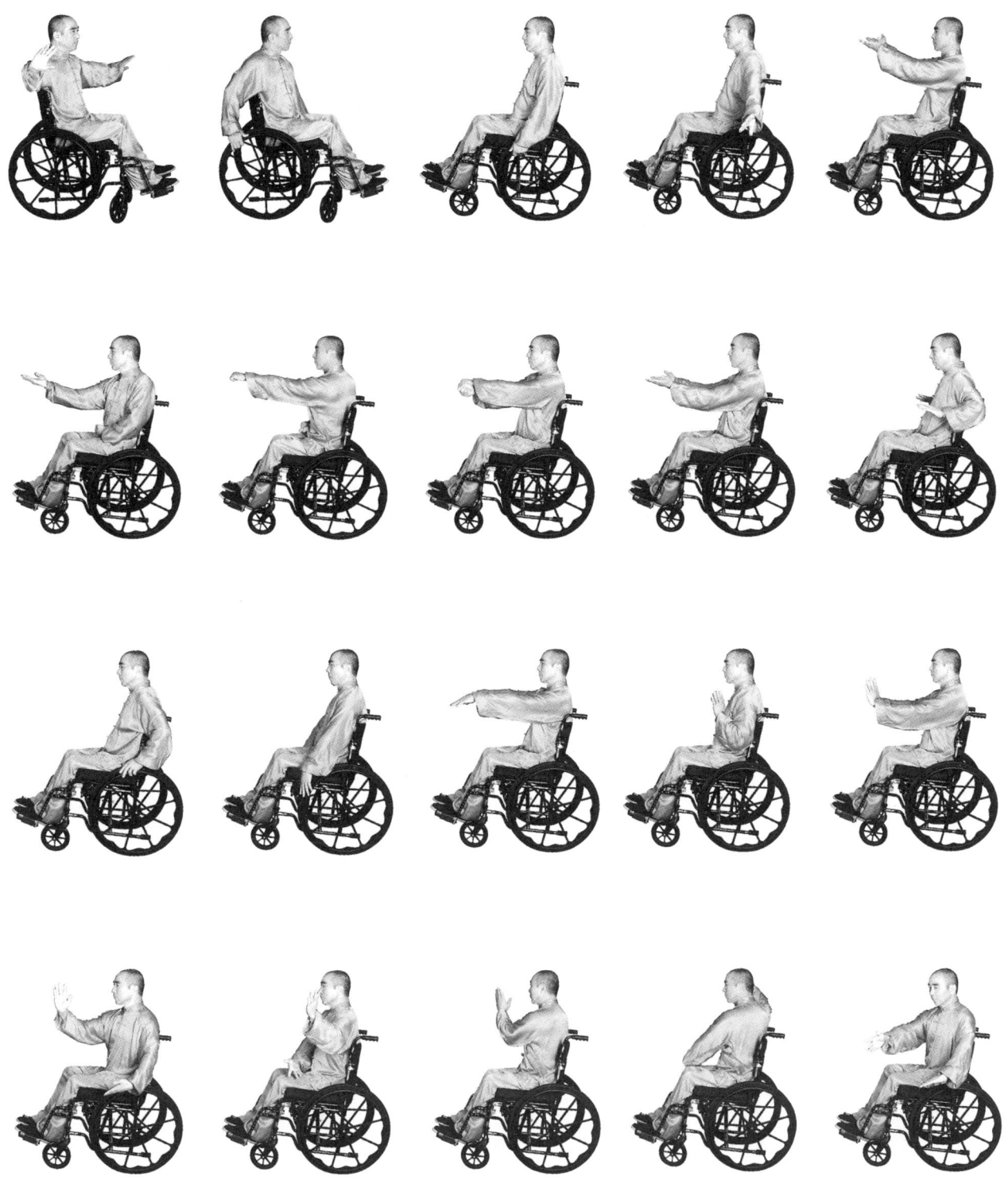

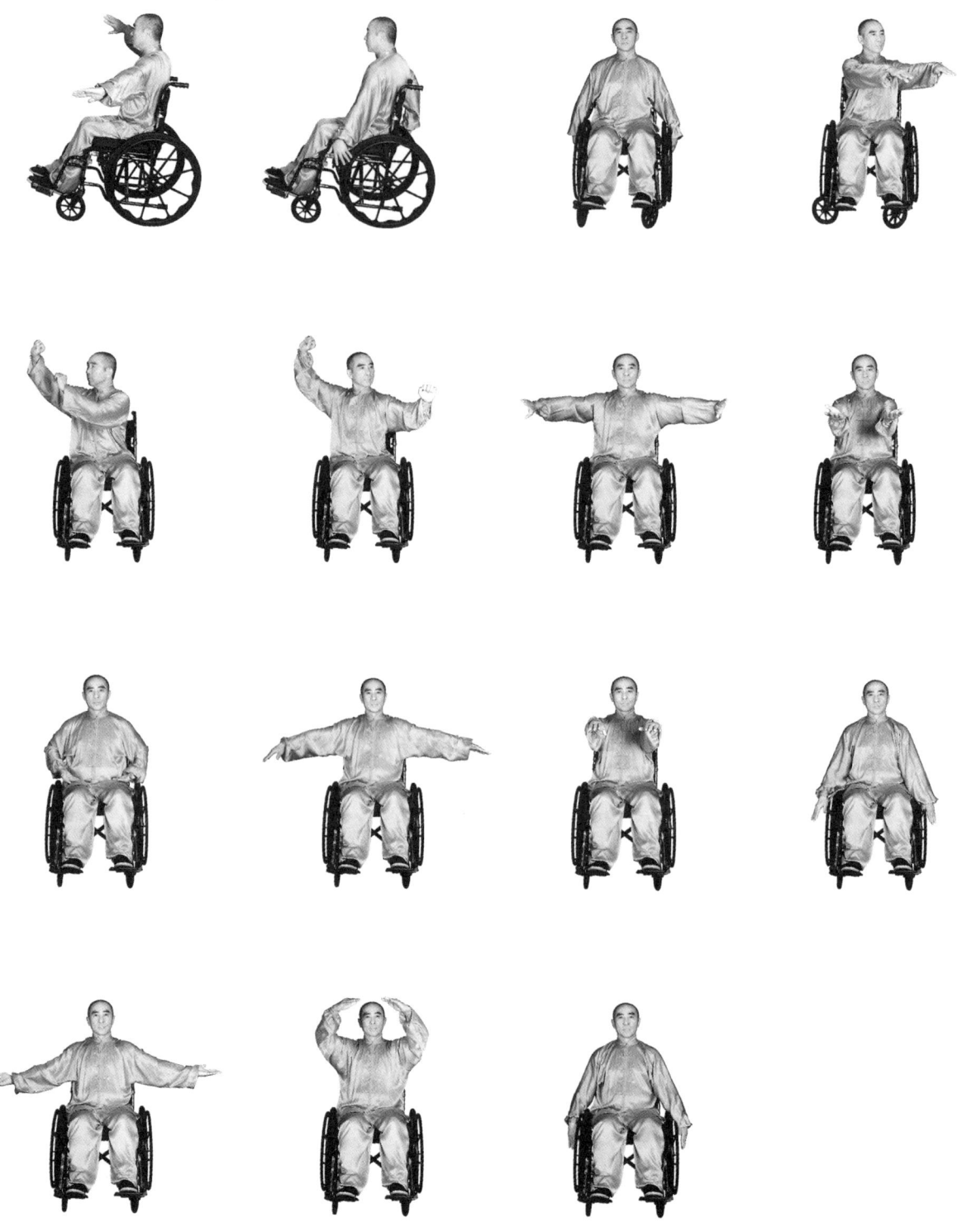

STANDING TAI CHI CHUAN

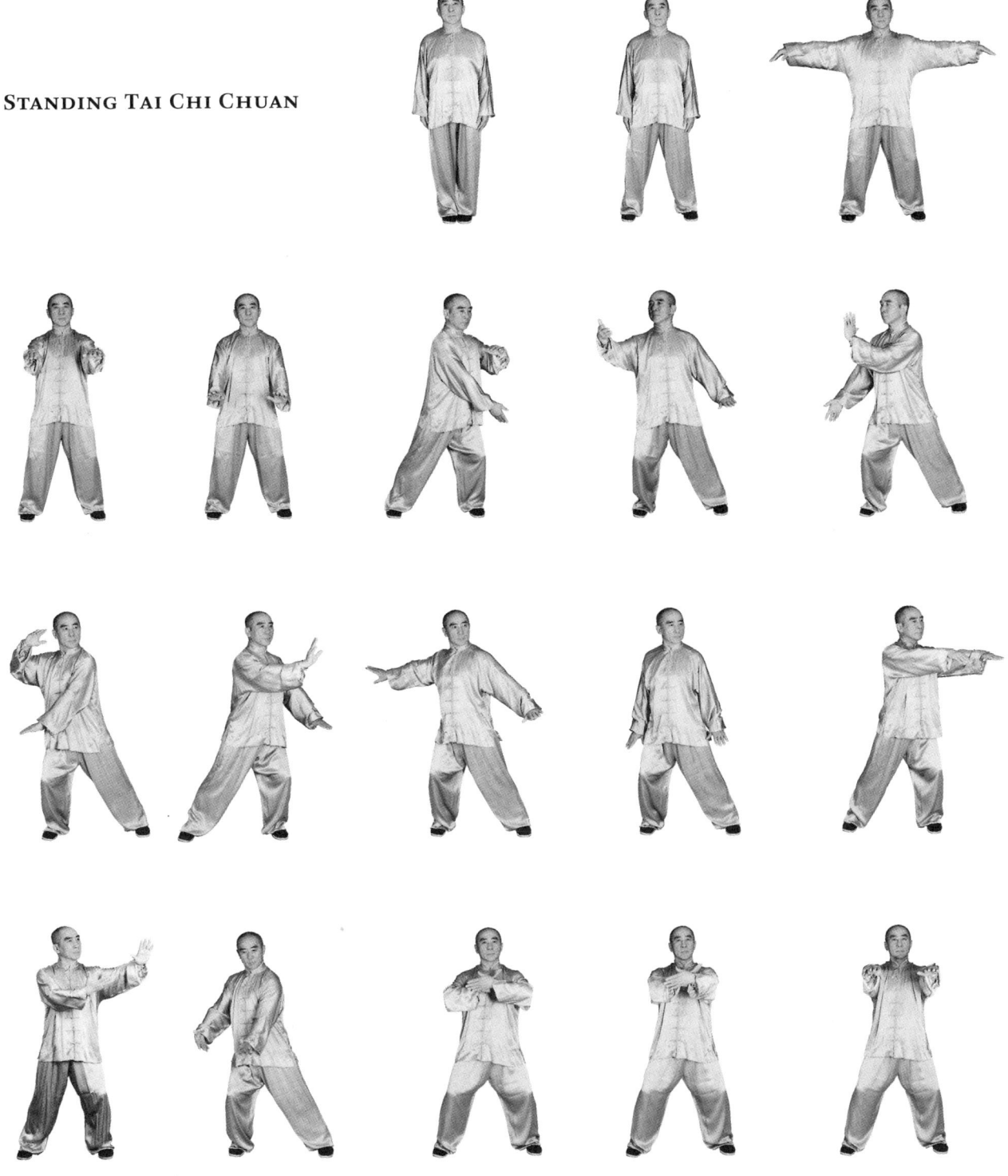

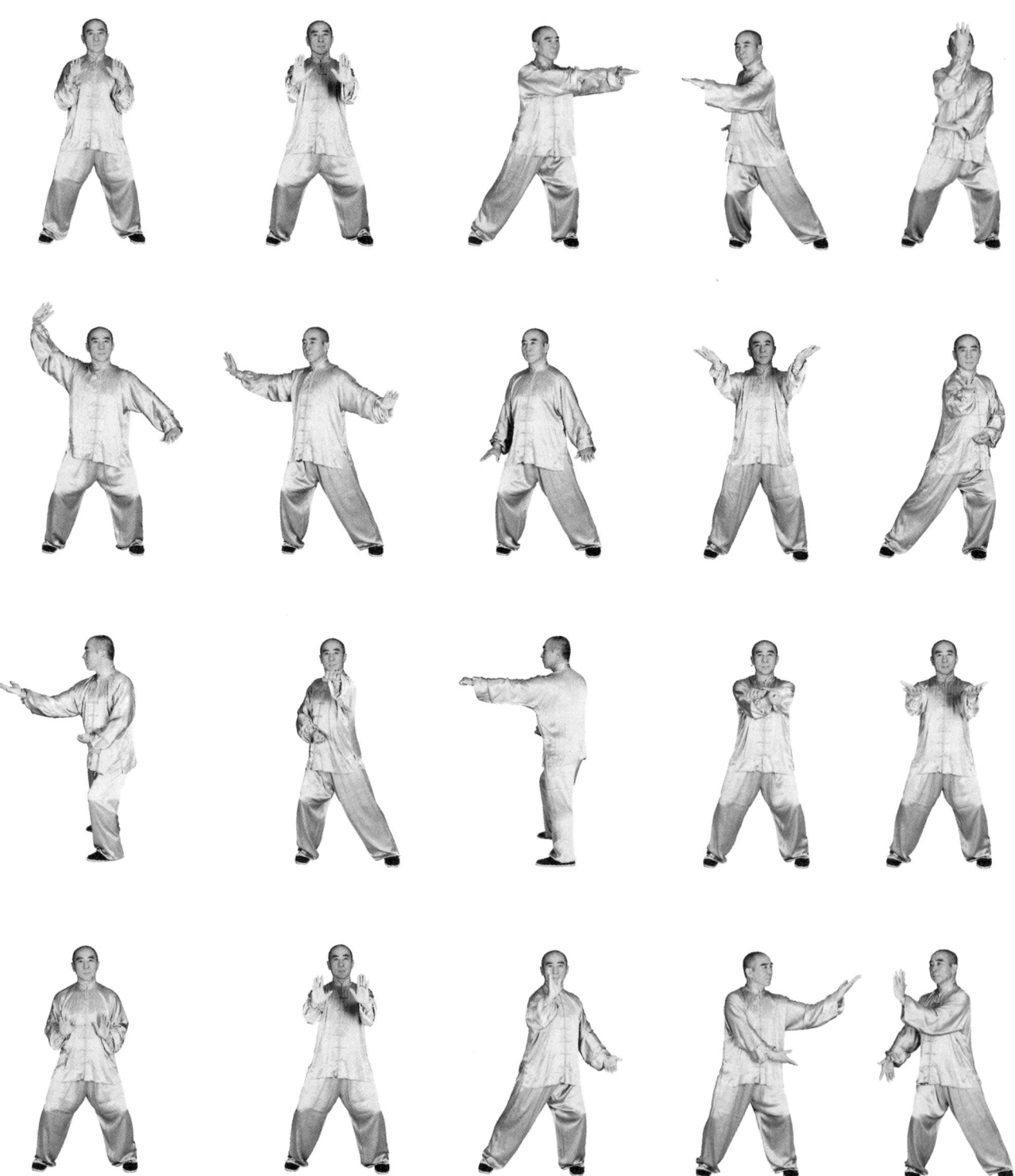

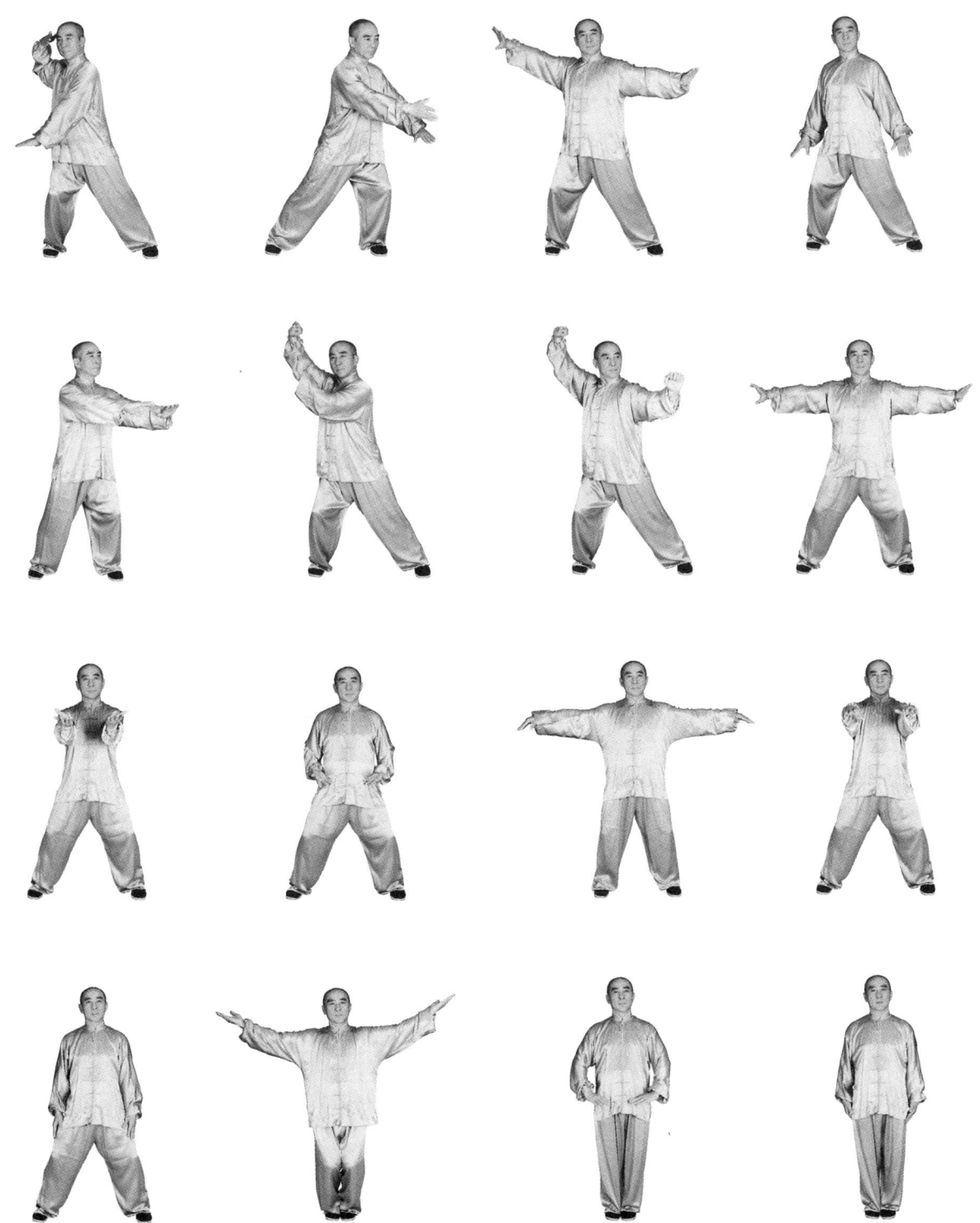

WALKING TAI CHI CHUAN

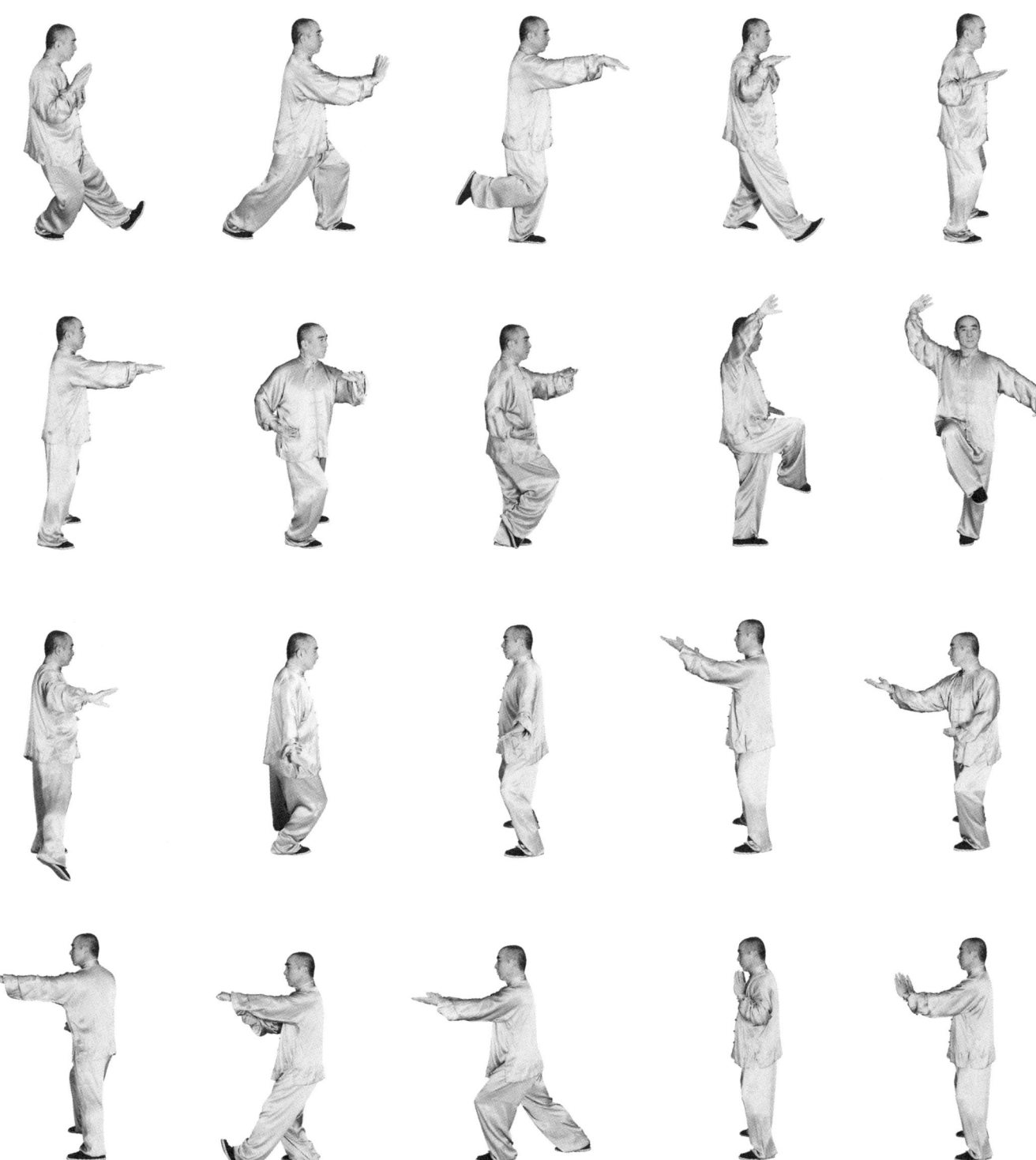

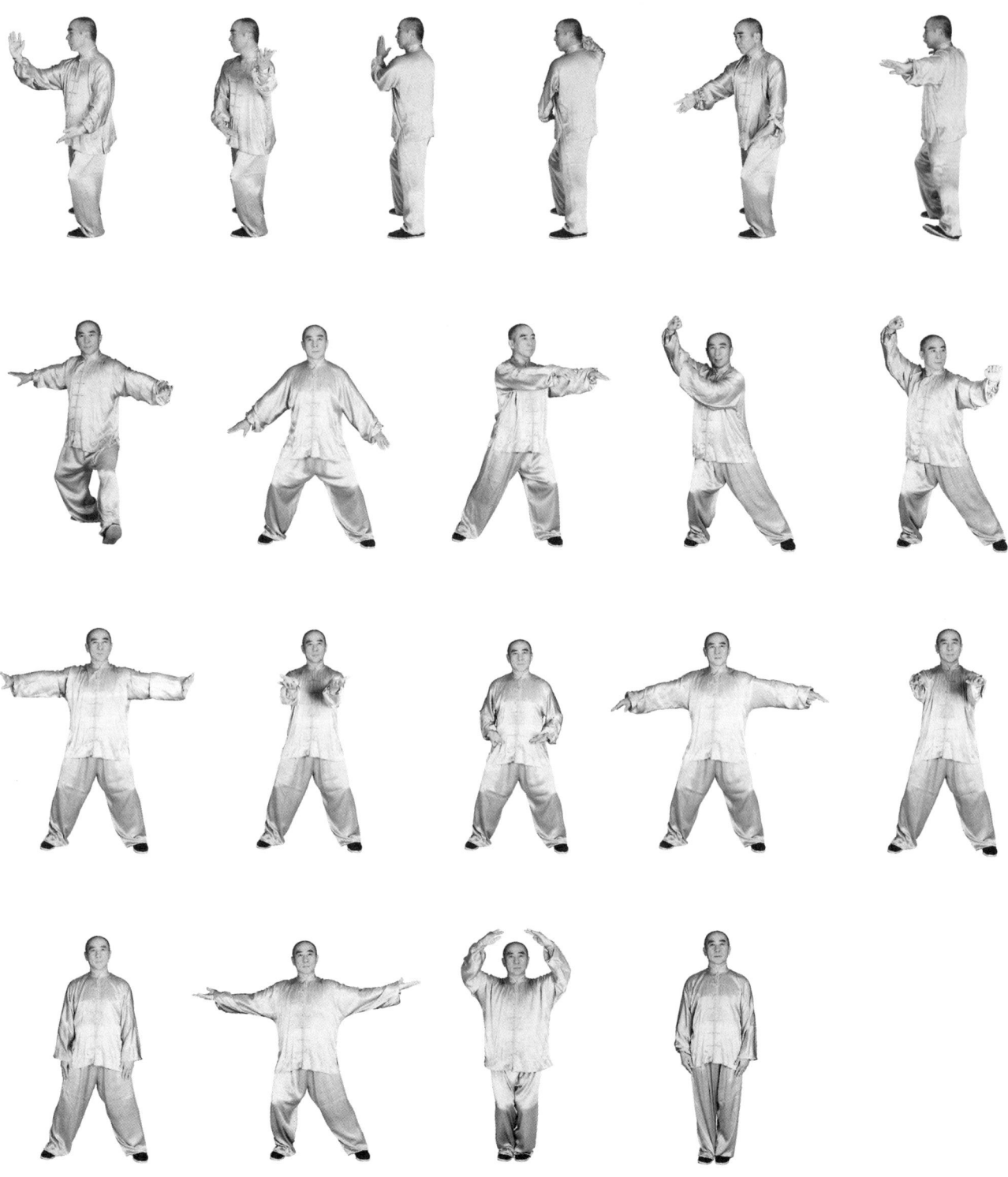

SEATED TAI CHI CHUAN

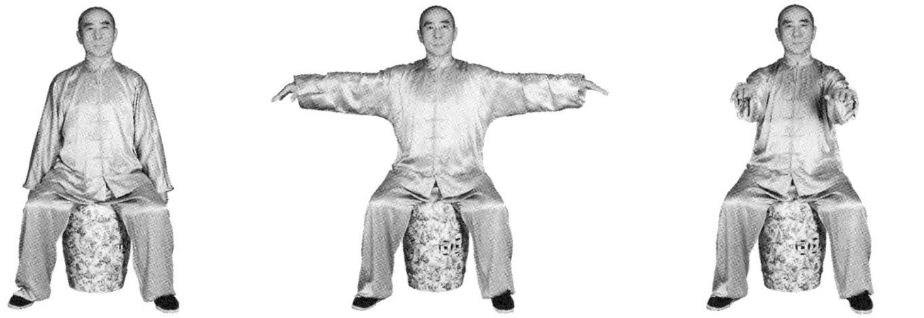

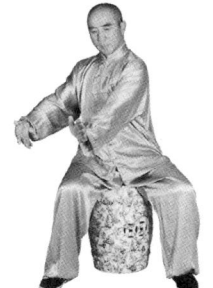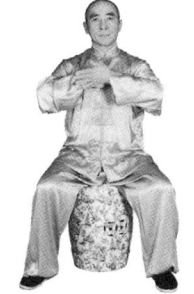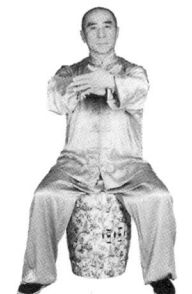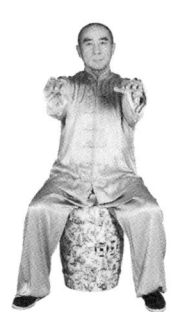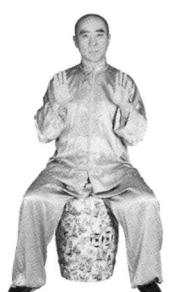

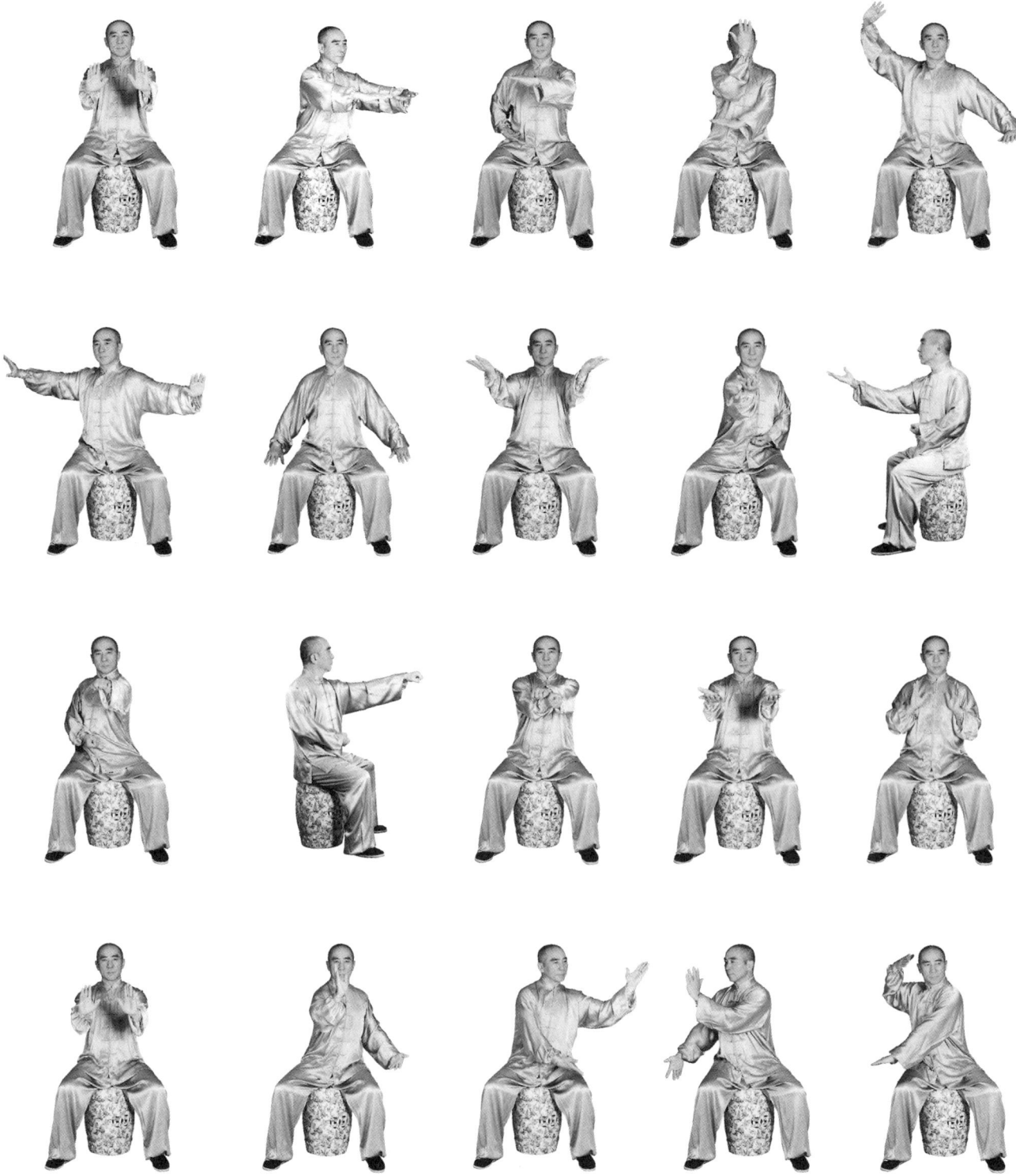

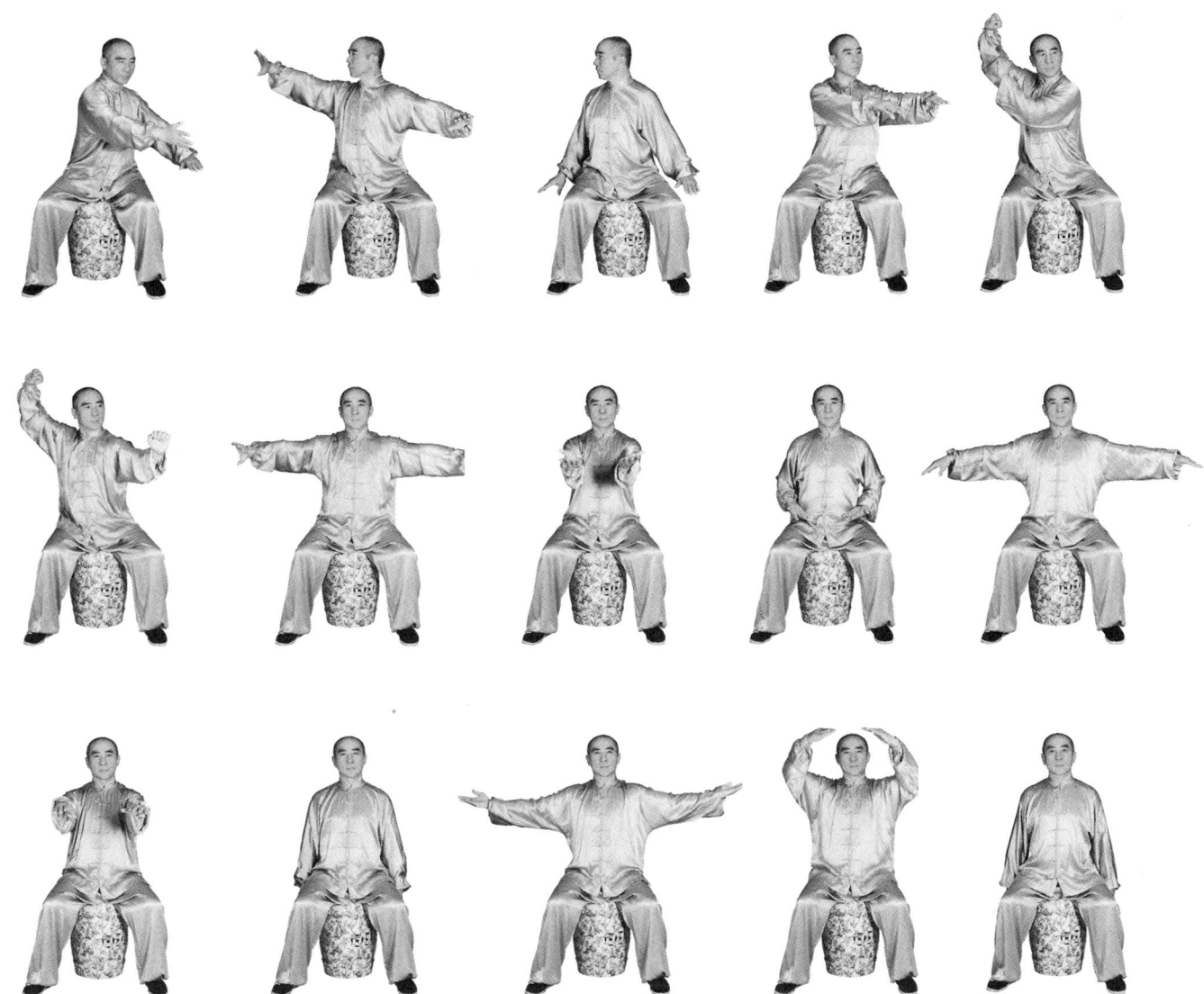

SINGLE-MOVE TAI CHI CHUAN

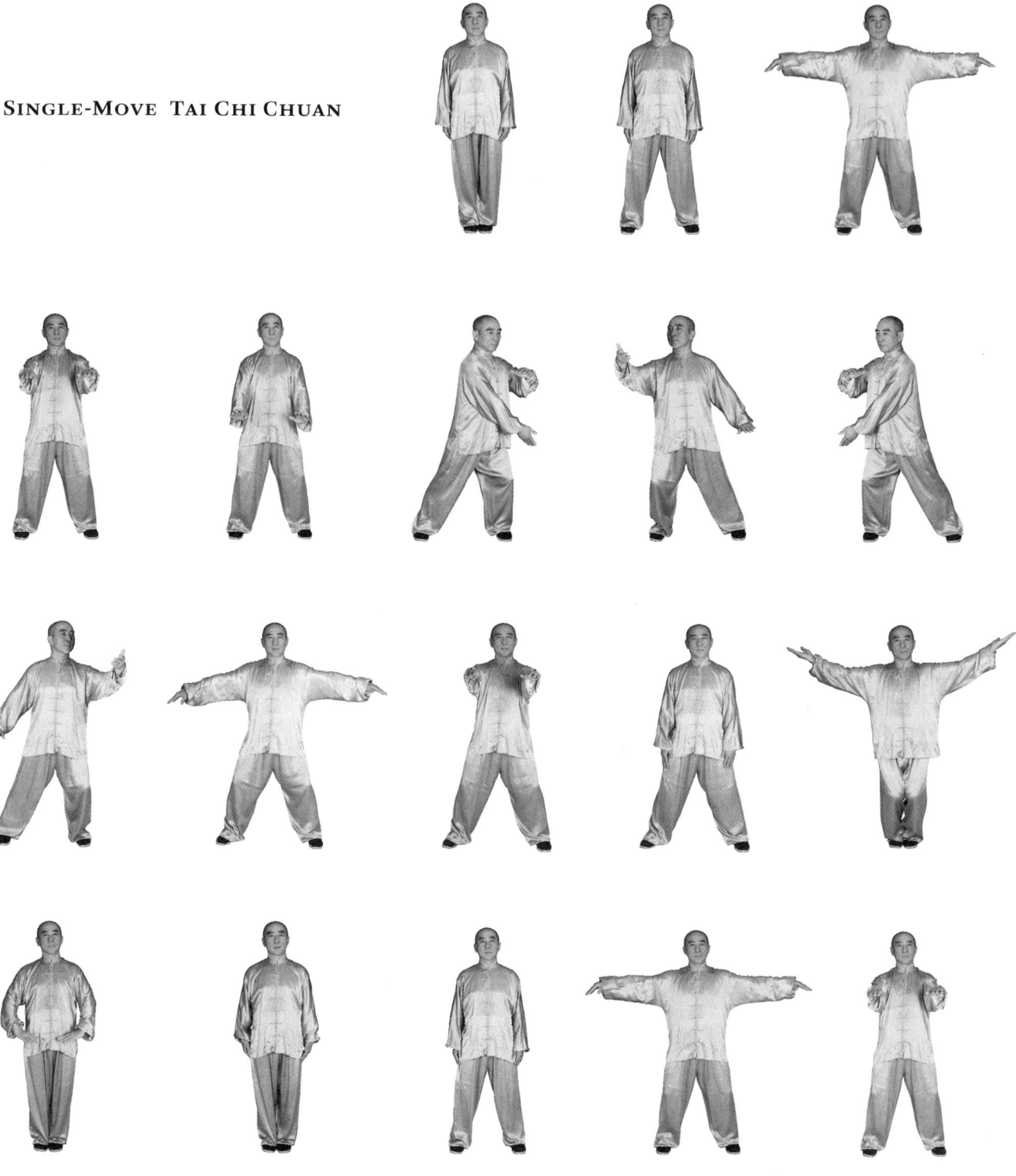

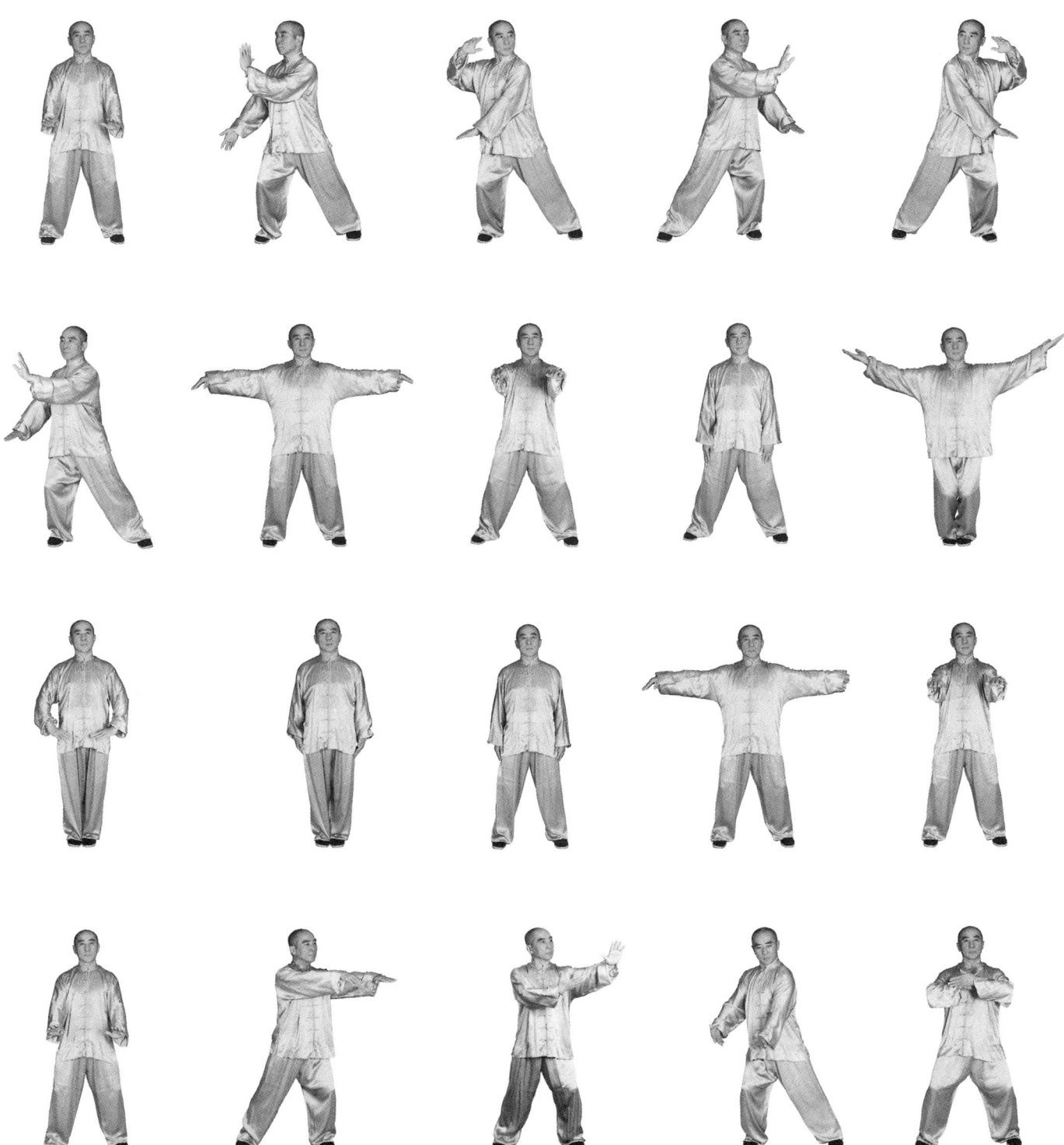

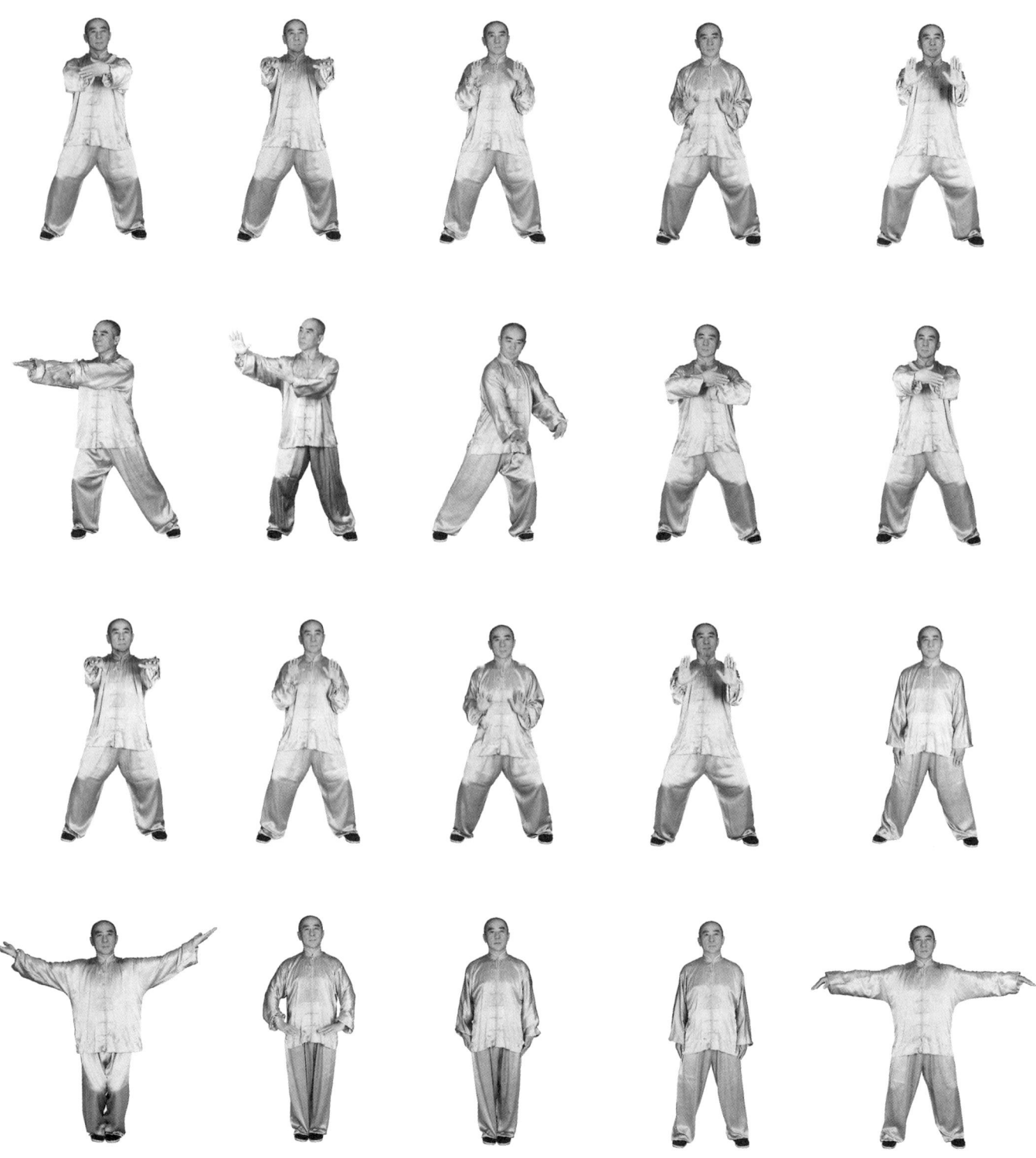

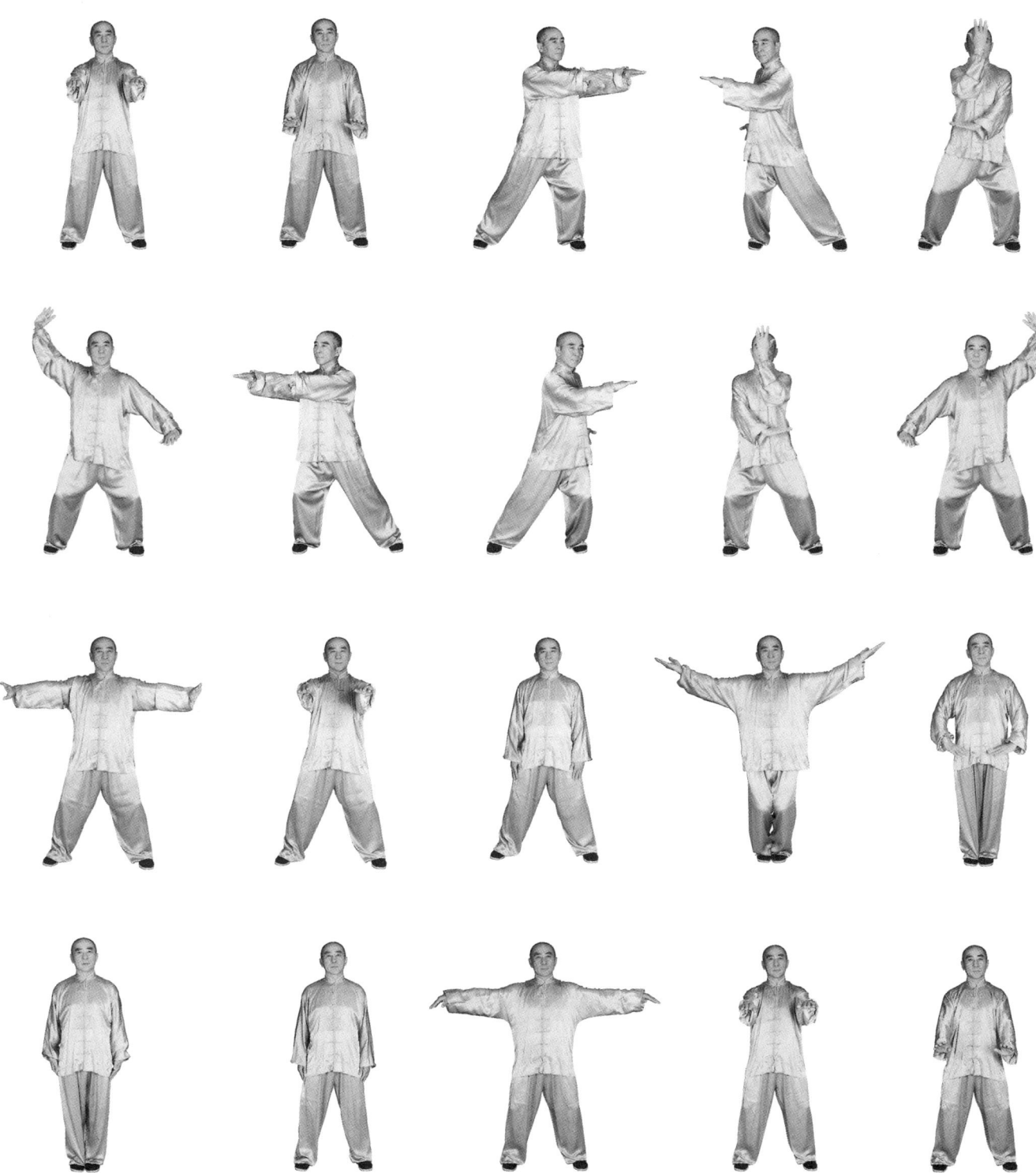

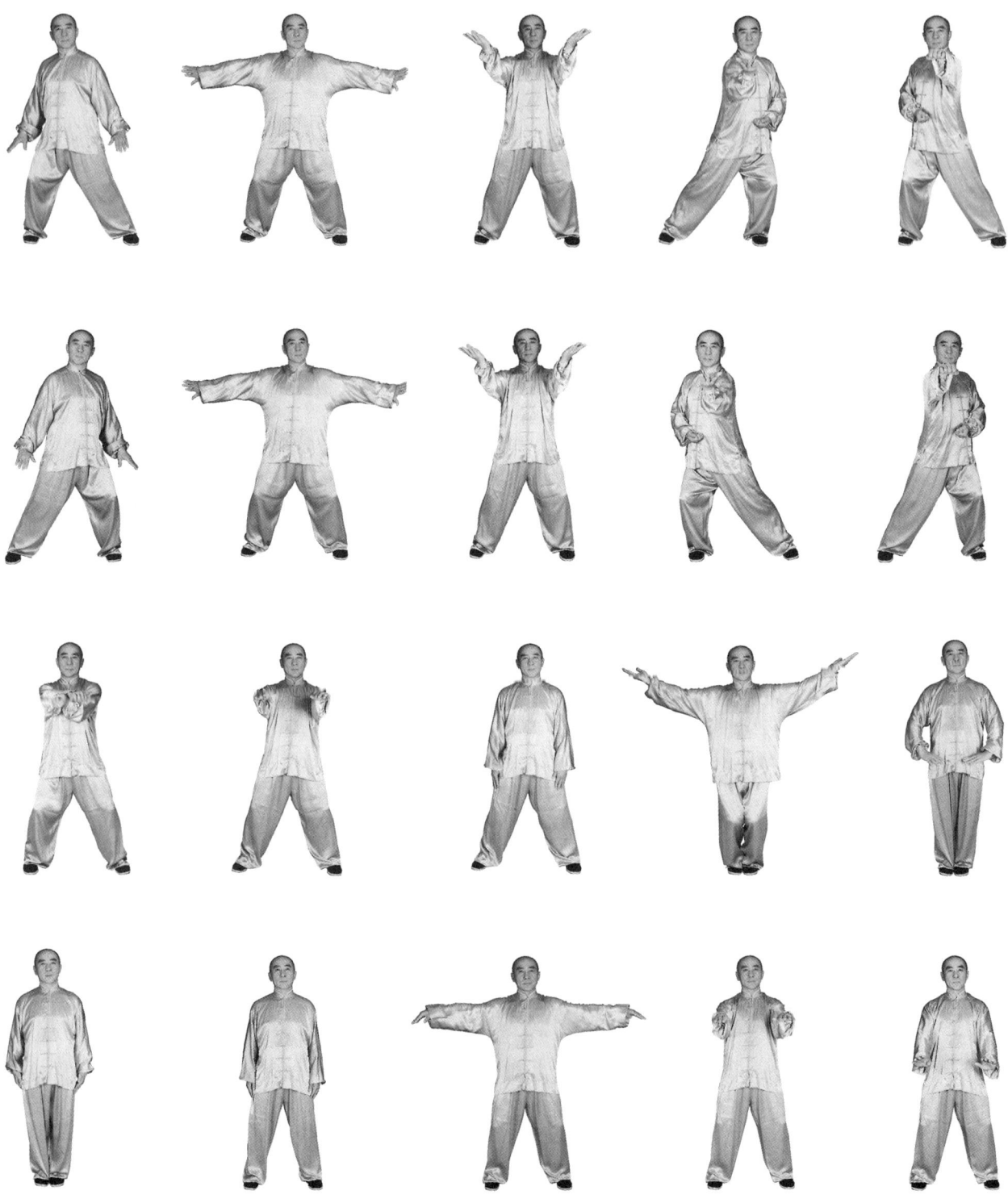

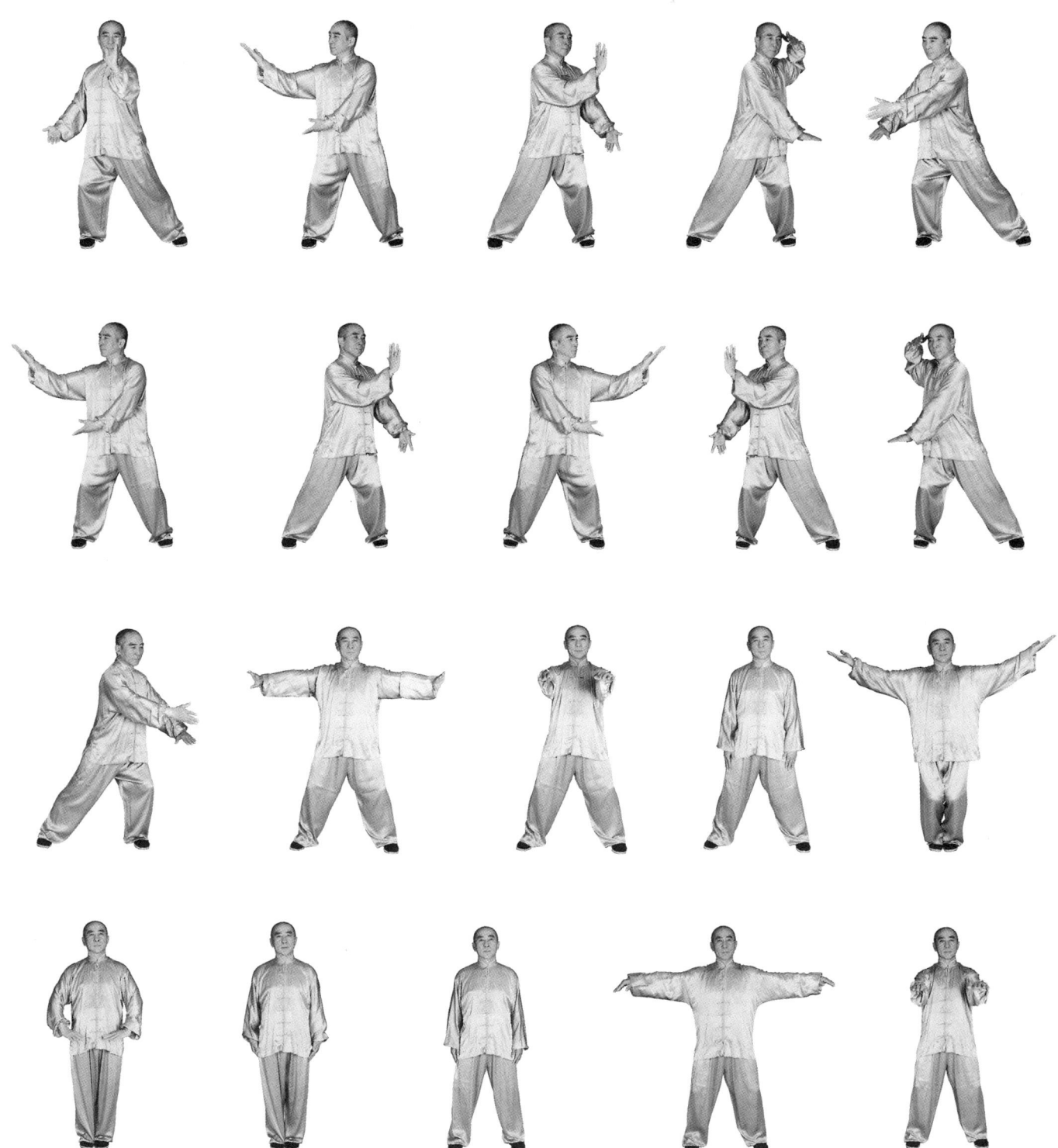

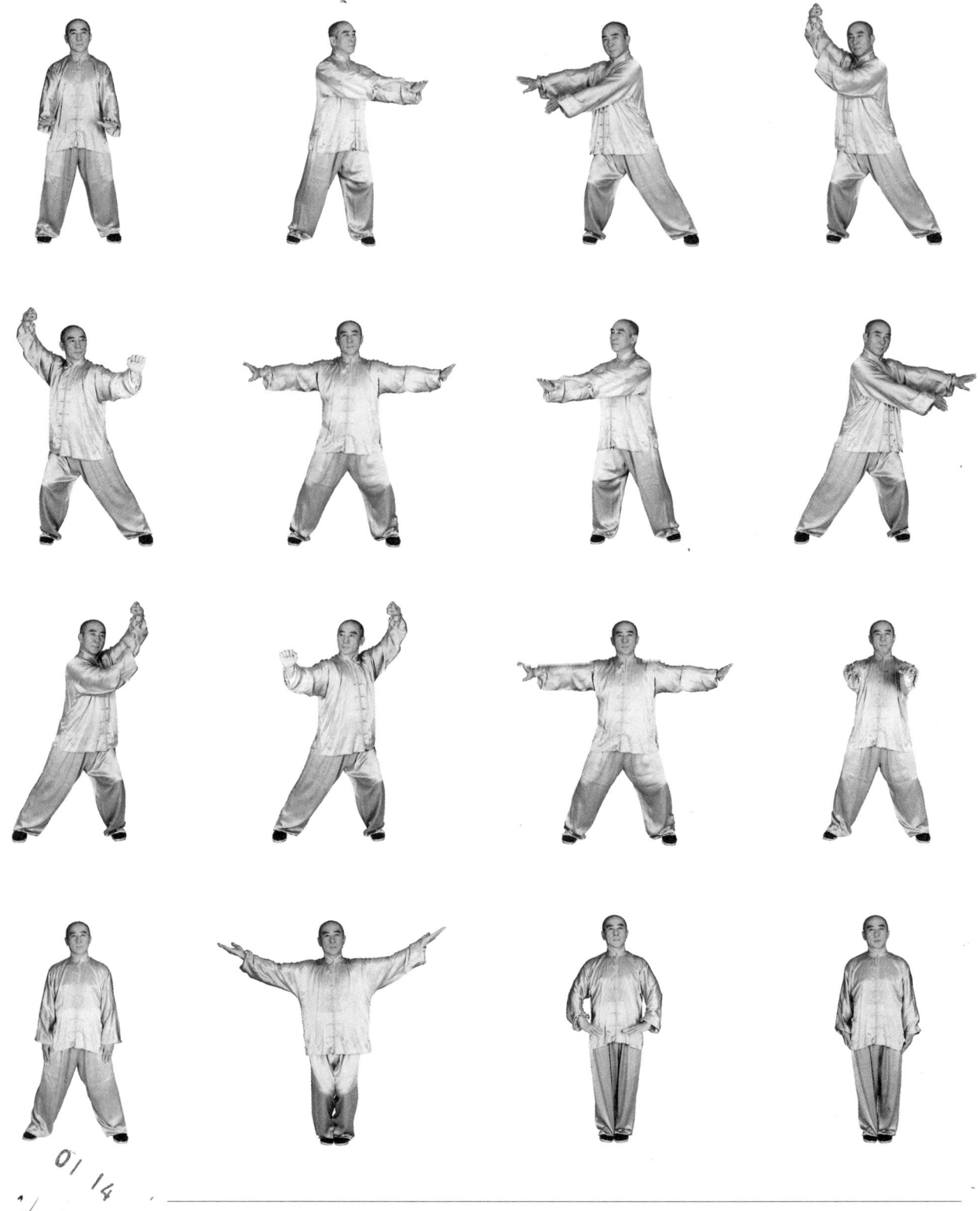

01 14